Air Fryer cookbook

Enjoy Mouth-Watering, Budget-Friendly, and Easy-To-Make Recipes. Fry, Bake, and Toast Every Meal You Desire In Minutes.

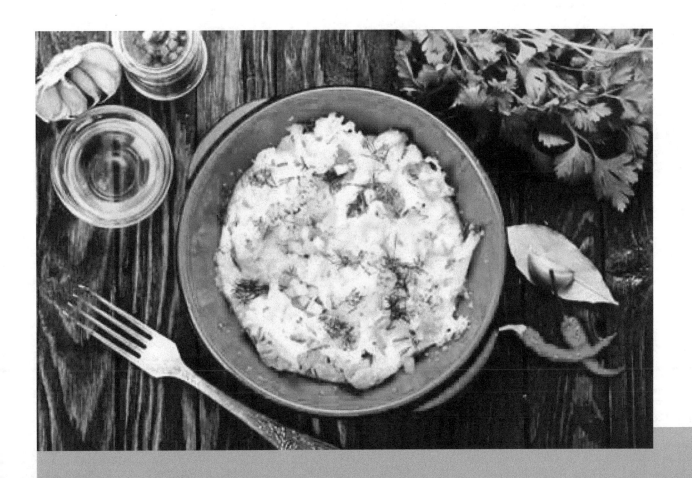

LAURA OWEN

Introduction

Air fryers are fundamentally scaled-down ledge convection ovens with a heating component over the food and a solid fan. As it creates heat, the fan circles the sight-seeing to enable the food to cook equitably and crispy. When contrasted with customary rotisserie foods, most air fried food surfaces have fundamentally the same as smash without utilizing a huge amount of oil or fat. Truth be told, we scarcely need to utilize any oil and the food despite everything that turns out crispy and scrumptious. Most food likewise turns out like it's flawlessly roasted in a convection oven with magnificent roasted flavors and surfaces. When breaded and splashed with oil, food becomes crunchy and fundamentally the same as what you would cook in a profound fryer.

We needed to tell everybody that air broiling isn't about re-heating solidified comfort foods. Indeed, it's incredible for heating remains and cooking snappy solidified bites. You can cook crisp, healthy, and healthy recipes in the air fryer. No doubt. Try not to JUDGE. Truly, we made a decision from the start, yet after our first straightforward feast for two individuals in under 20 minutes, we were snared and fixated and wild. Consequently, the formation of overly new and delightful recipes for the cookbooks.

Low-Fat Meals: Unarguably, the most basic advantage of the air fryer is its utilization of sight-seeing circulation to prepare nourishment fixings from all edges, in this manner wiping out the requirement for oil use. This makes it workable for individuals on a low-fat eating regimen to serenely prepare brilliantly sound suppers.

More beneficial Foods & Environment: Air fryers are intended to work without swelling oils and to deliver more advantageous nourishments with up to 80 percent less fat. This makes it simpler to get in shape since you can at present eat your seared dishes while moderating the calories and soaked fat. Doing that change to a more advantageous life is increasingly reachable by utilizing this apparatus. Your house is additionally freed of the fragrance that accompanies Pan-fried nourishments that regularly remains around the climate even a few hours after profound broiling.

Multipurpose Use: The air fryer empowers you to perform various tasks as it can prepare numerous dishes on the double. It is yours across the board machine that can flame broil, heat, fry, and meal those dishes that you love! You never again need numerous apparatuses for different occupations. It can do different employments separate machines will do. It can barbecue meat, cook veggies, and heat baked goods. It fills in as a viable substitution for your broiler, profound fryer, and stovetop.

Incredibly Safe: Remember how extra cautious you must be while tossing chicken or some different fixings into the profound fryer? You need to guarantee that the hot oil doesn't spill and consume your skin since it's in every case extremely hot. With your air fryer, you wouldn't have to stress over brunt skin from hot oil spillage. It does all the broiling and is protected. By the by, use cooking gloves while repositioning your fryer to maintain a strategic distance from dangers from the warmth.

Furthermore, keep your air fryer out of youngsters' compass.

Simple Clean Up: The Air Fryer leaves no oil and, along these lines, no wreckage. Tidy up time is agreeable since their oils spill to clean on dividers and floors, and no rejecting or scouring of the container. The Air fryer parts are made of non-stick material, which keeps nourishment from adhering to surfaces along these lines, making it difficult to clean. These parts are anything but difficult to clean and keep up. They are removable and dishwasher-sheltered too.

Spare Valuable Time: People who are on tight calendars can utilize the quickness of the air fryer to make tasty suppers. For occasions, you can make French fries in under 15 minutes and heat a cake inside 25 minutes. Inside minutes as well, you can appreciate fresh chicken fingers or brilliant fries. On the off chance that you are consistently in a hurry, the air fryer is perfect for you since you will invest less energy in the kitchen. It empowers you to deal with your rushed and occupied day by day life, filling your heart with joy increasingly sensible.

Prepare your fixings and put them into the crate, and afterward set your clock. The tourist goes to work, and when his work is finished, the clock goes off with a ding sound, showing that your nourishment is finished. You may even check your nourishment to perceive how it's advancing without upsetting the set time. When you pull out the container, the fryer will delay; when you place back the skillet, warming will proceed.

The Air fryer is a direct apparatus, with no collecting required and no confusion. It comprises three principle things; the cooking container, the skillet, and the primary fryer unit.

The Cooking Basket is the place you put your nourishment. It has a crate handle where you place your hand when taking care of the apparatus and prepared nourishment to forestall consumption or wounds when the air fryer is turned on. The bushel fits splendidly into the skillet. The pan gathers the nourishment remainders and overabundance oil and fits impeccably into the air fryer & then we have The Main Fryer Unit, which comprises numerous parts. Other helpful parts incorporate a rack, twofold flame broil layer, a bushel, and nourishment separators that make it conceivable to prepare various dishes immediately.

Contents

CONCLUSION

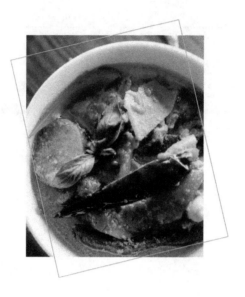

CHAPTER 1: WHAT IS AN AIR FRYER?

An air fryer utilizes the convection mechanism in cooking food. It circulates hot air through the use of a mechanical fan to cook the ingredients inside the fryer.

The process was named after the person who first explained it in 1912, French chemist Louis-Camille Maillard. The effect gives a distinctive flavor to browned foods, such as bread, biscuits, cookies, pan-fried meat, seared steaks, and many more.

The air fryer requires only a thin layer of oil for the ingredients to cook. It circulates hot air up to 392 degrees Fahrenheit. It's an innovative way of eliminating up to 80 percent of the oil that is traditionally used for frying different foods and preparing pastries.

You can find a dose of friendly features in air fryers, depending on the brand you're using. Most brands include a timer adjustment and temperature control setting to make cooking easier and precise. An air fryer comes with a cooking basket where you'll place the food. The basket is placed on top of a drip tray. Depending on the model you're using, you will either be prompted to shake the basket to distribute the oil evenly, or it automatically does the job via a food agitator.

This is perfect for home use, but if you're cooking for many people and you want to apply the same cooking technique, you can put your food items in specialized air crisper trays and cook them using a convection oven. An air fryer and convection oven apply the same technique in cooking, but an air fryer has a smaller built and produces less heat.

Directions Use Your Air Fryer

This appliance comes with a manual for easy assembly and as a handy guide for first-time users. Most brands also include a pamphlet of recipes to give your ideas about the wide range of dishes that you can create using this single kitchen appliance. Once you are ready to cook and you have all your ingredients ready, put them in the basket and insert them into the fryer. Other recipes will require you to preheat the air fryer before using it. Once the basket is in, set the temperature and timer and begin cooking.

You can use an air fryer for cooking food in a variety of ways. Once you get used to the basics, you can try its other features, such as advanced baking and using air fryer dehydrators.

Here are some of the cooking techniques that you can do with this single appliance:

Fry: You can omit oil in cooking, but a little amount adds crunch and flavor to your food. You can add oil to the ingredients while mixing or lightly spray the food with oil before cooking. You can use most kinds of oils, but many users prefer peanut, olive, sunflower, and canola oils.

Roast: You can produce the same quality of roasted foods as the ones cooked in a conventional roaster in a faster manner. This is recommended to people who need to come up with a special dish but do not have much time to prepare.

Bake: There are baking pans suited for this appliance that you can use to bake bread, cookies, and other pastries. It only takes around 15 to 30 minutes to get your baked goodies done.

Grill: It effectively grills your food easily and without a mess. You only need to shake the basket halfway through the cooking process or flip the ingredients once or twice, depending on the instructions. To make it easier, you can put the ingredients in a grill pan or grill layer with a handle, which other models include in the package, or you can also buy one as an added accessory.

There are many kinds of foods that you can cook using an air fryer, but there are also certain types that are not suited for it. Avoid cooking ingredients, which can be steamed, like beans and carrots. You also cannot fry foods covered in heavy batter in this appliance.

Aside from the above mentioned, you can cook most kinds of ingredients using an air fryer. You can use it for cooking foods covered in light flour or bread crumbs. You can cook a variety of vegetables in the appliance, such as cauliflower, asparagus, zucchini, kale, peppers, and corn on the cob. You can also use it for cooking frozen foods, and home-prepared meals by following a different set of instructions for these purposes.

An air fryer also comes with another useful feature - the separator. It allows you to cook multiple dishes at a time. Use the separator to divide ingredients in the pan or basket. You have to make sure that all ingredients have the same temperature setting so that everything will cook evenly at the same time.

Cleaning and maintenance of Air Fryer

Along with careful cleaning, an electric appliance also needs constant maintenance. To ensure personal safety, all the components of the product have to be checked at least once a week. It is important to examine the power cord and its functionality. In case of the following anomalies, contact the Instant pot support team immediately:

1. If the power plug and cord show any damage, deformation, discoloration, and expansion.

2. If a certain portion of the power plug and the cord feels hotter than usual.

3. If the instant pot shows abnormal heating or emits a burnt smell.

4. If the cooker produces any abnormal sounds or vibrations when its power is on.

Caution: Unplug the device immediately when you find any such anomalies. Do not try to repair anything by yourself. Contact the support team and discuss the issue in detail.

CHAPTER 2: BENEFITS OF THE AIR FRYER

Healthy cooking, time saver, easy of use, easy of clean up, versatility

Healthier Cooking: add an air fryer to your kitchen gadgets if you're looking to cut down on calories but don't want to lose flavor or taste. Although deep frying food can use up to three cups of oil, most air fryers use only one cubic cubicle. They use air and minimum oil to heat and cook the food. The effect is crispy meals with fewer calories than conventional deep frying.

Time-saving kitchen utensil: This takes some time to pre-heat oil and ovens. An air fryer can achieve a temperature in a matter of minutes. In an air fryer, food cooks quicker too.

Easy to use: Many air fryers come with presets to cook popular dishes by pressing a button. Because cooking is done within the air fryer, and the temperature is set automatically, walking away from it is healthy and not worried about grease fires.

Fast Cleaning: A large quantity of oil is used for deep frying. In addition to splattering while frying, there is leftover oil that can be difficult (and annoying) to dispose of after everything is cooked. There is no oil to get rid of since minimum oil is being used. The air fryer parts are a safe dishwasher making it easy to clean up.

Low-calorie food: Hot air fryers add little calories to food. Calories can be helpful at certain times, but too much is never a good option. This cooking tool avoids all of these unhealthy fats and keeps your food healthy at all times. Lowering calories can help you lose weight and help you lose weight if you have problems.

Little oil: The use of additional oils besides the food oil, which is fried, can be completely avoided. Hot air fryers work best when the food is dry and ungreased. This is much healthier than soaking food in oil using a traditional tempura pan.

Burning oil produces substances that are medically proven to cause cancer and cardiovascular problems such as heart failure. Furthermore, saving on oil purchases and saving money is not a bad thing.

Tips and Tricks of using Air Fryer

1. PRE-HEAT YOUR AIR FRYER... for a proper, it normal practice that any cooking item should be pre-heated. Often I do it, sometimes I don't do it, and my meal is still good. And in case your air fryer is without a pre-heat feature, simply turn it to the desired temperature and allow it to run for about 3 minutes before bringing adding the food.

2. USE OIL FOR FOODS COOKED IN THE AIR FRYER... I like using oils for certain foods to make them crisp, but some foods don't always need it.

3. DON'T OVERLOAD THE BASKET: If you want your fried food to turn out to be fresh, you'll want to make sure you don't congest the refrigerator. Placing too much food in the bowl will keep the food from stretching and browning. Cook your food in containers or invest in a larger air fryer to make sure this doesn't happen.

4. SHAKE THE BASKET DURING FRYING, WINGS, AND OTHER COOKING. When frying small items such as chicken wings and French fries, shake the basket every few minutes to ensure uniform cooking, sometimes, instead of throwing, use a pair of silicone kitchen pins to flip over larger items

5. SPRAY HALFWAY THROUGH COOKING: I find that spraying oil halfway through cooking is best done on most foods. Coated food items are to be sprayed. Additionally, spray some dried flour spots that still surface halfway through the rain.

6. WATER / BREAD IN THE BASE STOPS WHITE SMOKE: If it is time to fry a greasy food in your air fryer, don't be shocked to see some white smoke pouring out of the machine. To solve the problem, just dump a little (about 2Tbsp) of water in the bottom of the container, the smoke stops and the food continues to cook.

Some people place a slice of bread at the bottom of the unit to blot the grease when preparing items that can spread large amounts of grease, such as bacon.

7. LOOKOUT FOR THE SMALL LIGHT ITEMS IN THE AIR FRYER: most of the Air Fryer unit has a powerful fan at the top of the unit.

8. ADJUST THE TEMPERATURE: Most times, you want to turn the heat of the Air Fryer to the highest temperature to encourage it to work but be careful as some foods will dry out easily. A proper way is to adjust the temperature and time from how long you would usually do it in the oven. I like to go down 30 degrees and cut the time by about 20 percent. For starters, if you baked brownies at 350 degrees Fahrenheit in the oven for 20 minutes, cut the Air Fryer to 320 degrees and cook for about 16 minutes.

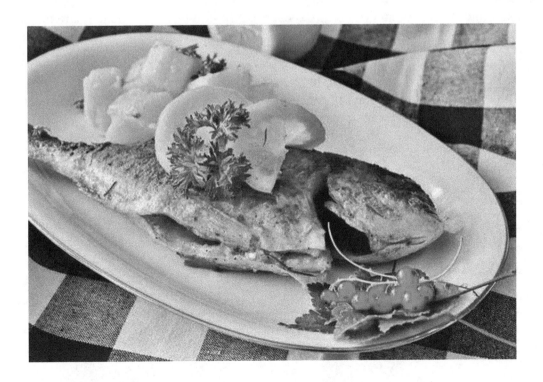

CHAPTER 3: OTHER TIPS USING THE AIR FRYER

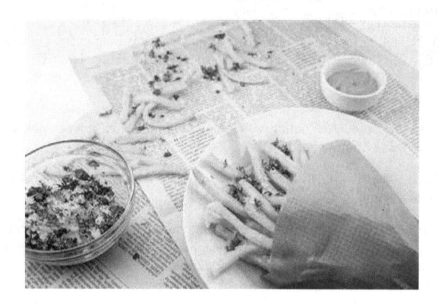

Air fryers are designed to be super easy to use. Here's a little guide to get you started.

Choose a recipe

Choose a recipe that you can cook in your air fryer. Remember that most foods that you cook in your microwave or oven, or on the stovetop, can be prepared in the air fryer – except for those recipes that have a lot of fat or liquids. You can use my air fryer cookbook to help you find suitable recipes.

Prepare the air fryer

Read through the recipe to the end, so you know what accessories you need for cooking. Some recipes call for using the basket, rack, or rotisserie that comes with the air fryer. Other recipes use cake or muffin pans that you can insert into the air fryer. Just be sure these pans fit into the fryer and are safe to use.

Prepare the ingredients

Gather the ingredients for the recipe and prep them according to the instructions. When prepped, put the ingredients into the air fryer or in the basket, rack, or pans within the air fryer. Use parchment baking paper or a light mist of oil spray to prevent food from sticking.

Never crowd food in the air fryer or over-fill. Food that is crowded in the air fryer won't cook evenly and can be raw and under-cooked. If you're preparing for a crowd, you may have to cook more than one batch.

Setting the temperature and time

Check the recipe for the correct temperature and time setting. You can set it manually, r you can use the digital setting for the temperature and time needed for the recipe. Most air fryers also have preset functions that make it easy to set according to each recipe.

Check food during cooking

Many air fryer recipes require you to check the food while it's cooking so that it cooks evenly and doesn't over-cook. All you need to do is shake, flip, or toss the food to distribute it. Or for some recipes, you'll need to turn the food about halfway through when cooking so that it cooks and crisps thoroughly all the way through.

Cleaning the air fryer

Once the food is cooked, remove, and unplug the air fryer. Let it cool completely before cleaning. Follow the instructions that come with the fryer for proper cleaning. Never scrub or use abrasive cleaners when cleaning the fryer or the fryer accessories. What air fryer should you use?

The recipes in my book can be used with any model of an air fryer. This includes oven-style fryers that have horizontal racks or fryers that have a basket and handle.

My recipes were developed for my air fryer – it only has a temperature and timer setting. But you'll able to make any of the recipes in my book even if your air fryer has preset functions or multiple functions for baking, broiling, and roasting. Choose a function that matches my recipe or use the manual setting if you're unsure.

Using the basket or rack

Some models of air fryers use a round basket where foods are cooked while other models will have layered racks that fit into a square cooking space, much like a small oven. My recipes can be used for both baskets and racks.

Keep an eye on timing

You will find that air fryers cook at different temperatures depending on what model you have. This is why it's important to check on foods during the cooking process, so you don't over or undercook them. If you've cut back on quantities in some of my recipes, be sure to cut the cooking time down accordingly. Remember, my hints are just recommendations to guide you as you use your air fryer.

Using oil sprays

Most of my recipes in this book use oil spray – I use PAM. However, you can use any brand you want. Or make your own by merely putting olive oil into a small spray bottle. Use a small amount of oil and spray over the basket and trays to prevent food from sticking. Some of my recipes require you to spray the food with oil directly.

Function Keys

- **Button / Play/Pause Button**

This Play/Pause button allows you to pause during the middle of the cooking so you can shake the air fryer basket or flip the food to ensure it cooks evenly.

- **-/+ Button /Minus/Plus Button**

This button is used to change the time or temperature.

- **Keep Warm**

This function keeps your food warm for 30 minutes.

- **Food Presets**

This button gives you the ability to cook food without second-guessing. The time and temperature are already set, so new users find this setting useful.

- **Roast or Broil**

You can roast or broil with this setting. When using a conventional oven, you need to brown the meat before roasting. You can skip this step when cooking with an air fryer.

- **Dehydrate**

This setting cooks and dries food at a low temperature for a few hours. With this option, you can create your beef jerky or dried fruit.

CHAPTER 4: BREAKFAST

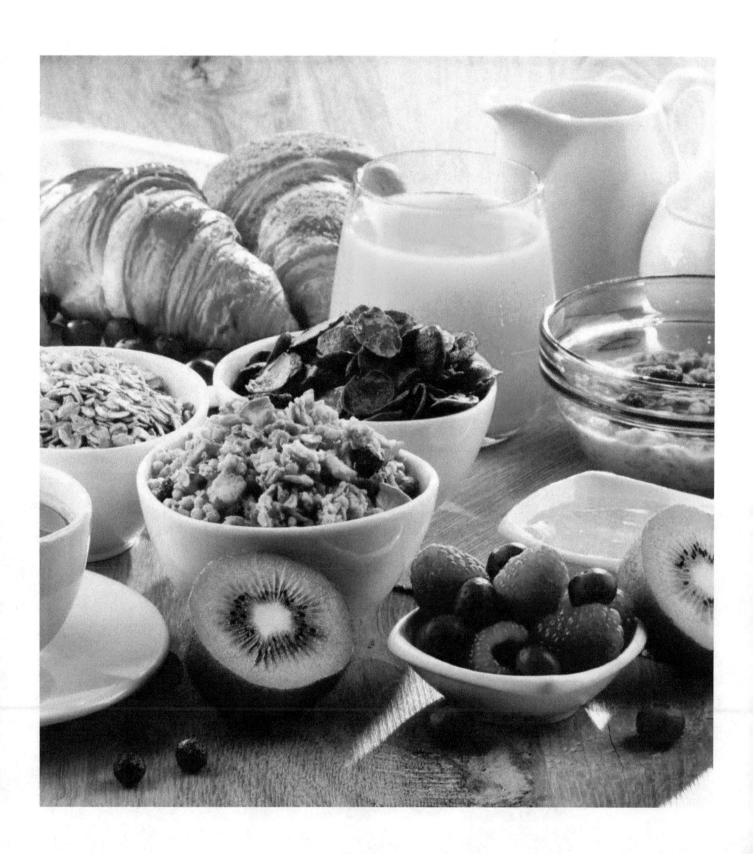

1. BREAKFAST EGG TOMATO
A Perfect and Classic Recipe for Family Breakfast

Easy

24 minutes

Breakfast

2 Servings

INGREDIENTS

2 eggs
2 large fresh tomatoes
1 tsp fresh parsley
Pepper
Salt

COOKING STEPS

1. Preheat the air fryer to 325 F.

2. Cut off the top of a tomato and spoon out the tomato innards.

3. Break the egg in each tomato, place it in the air fryer basket, and cook for 24 minutes.

4. Season with parsley, pepper, and salt.

5. Serve and enjoy.

Nutrition: Calories 255, Fat 16 g, Carbohydrates 8 g, Sugar 4.2 g, Protein 21 g.

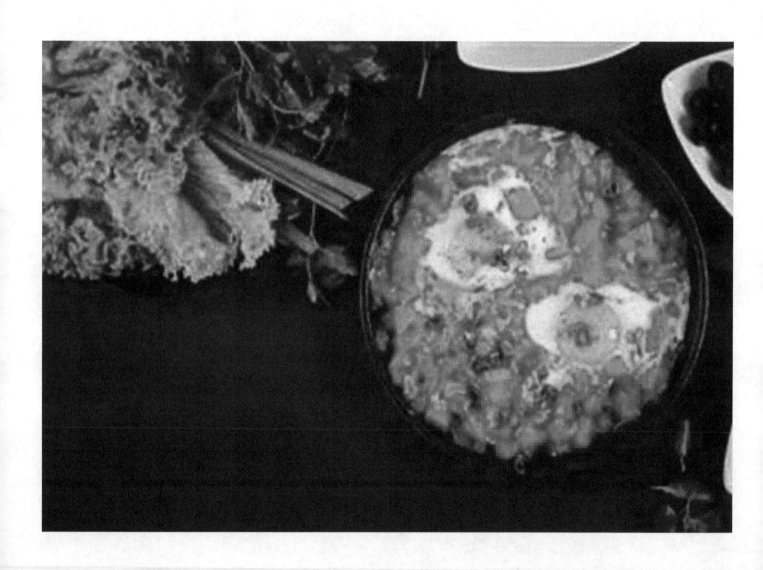

2. MUSHROOM LEEK FRITTATA
A Perfect and Classic Recipe for Family Breakfast

Easy

32 minutes

Breakfast

4 Servings

INGREDIENTS

6 eggs
6 oz. mushrooms, sliced
1 cup leeks, sliced
Salt

COOKING STEPS

1. Preheat the air fryer to 325 F.

2. Spray air fryer baking dish with cooking spray and set aside.

3. Heat another pan over medium heat. Spray pan with cooking spray.

4. Add mushrooms, leeks, and salt in a pan sauté for 6 minutes.

5. Break eggs in a bowl and whisk well.

6. Transfer sautéed mushroom and leek mixture into the prepared baking dish.

7. Pour egg over mushroom mixture.

8. Place dish in the air fryer and cook for 32 minutes.

9. Serve and enjoy.

Nutrition: Calories 255, Fat 16 g, Carbohydrates 8 g, Sugar 4.2 g, Protein 21 g.

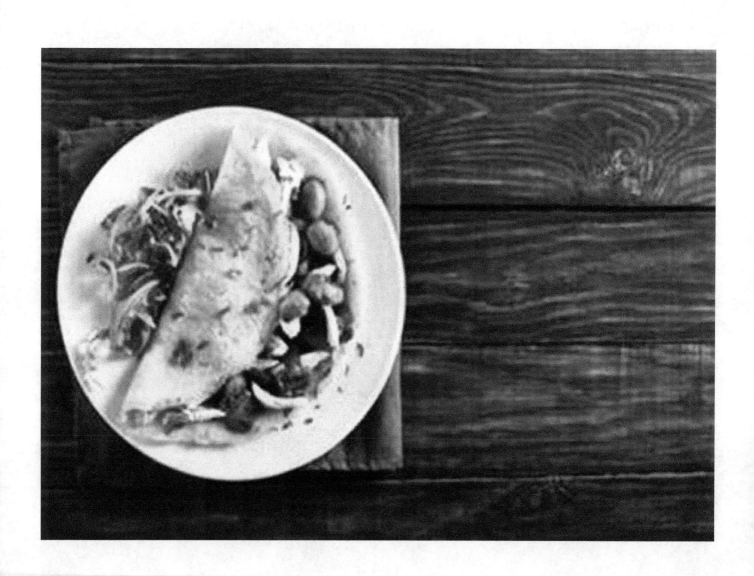

3. PERFECT BREAKFAST FRITTATA

A Perfect and Classic Recipe for Family Breakfast

Easy

32 minutes

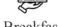
Breakfast

2 Servings

INGREDIENTS

3 eggs

2 tbsp. parmesan cheese, grated

2 tbsp. sour cream

1/2 cup bell pepper, chopped

1/4 cup onion, chopped

1/2 tsp pepper

1/2 tsp salt

COOKING STEPS

1. Add eggs to a mixing bowl and whisk with the remaining ingredients.

2. Spray air fryer baking dish with cooking spray.

3. Pour egg mixture into the prepared dish, place it in the air fryer, and cook at 350 F for 5 minutes.

4. Serve and enjoy.

Nutrition: Calories 277, Fat 15.2 g, Carbohydrates 6 g, Sugar 2.6 g, Protein 18.2 g.

4. INDIAN CAULIFLOWER

A Perfect and Classic Recipe for Family Breakfast

 Easy

 20 minutes

 Breakfast

 2 Servings

INGREDIENTS

3 cups cauliflower florets

2 tbsp. water

2 tsp fresh lemon juice

½ tbsp. ginger paste

1 tsp chili powder

¼ tsp turmeric

½ cup vegetable stock

Pepper

Salt

COOKING STEPS

1. Add all ingredients into the air fryer-baking dish and mix well.

2. Place dish in the air fryer and cook at 400 F for 10 minutes.

3. Stir well and cook at 360 F for 10 minutes more.

4. Stir well and serve.

Nutrition: Calories 49, Fat 0.5 g, Carbohydrates 9 g, Sugar 3 g, Protein 3 g.

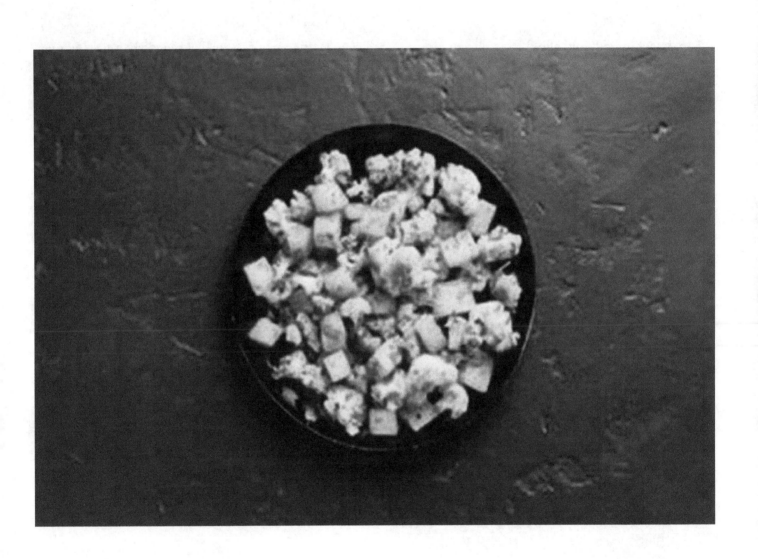

5. ZUCCHINI SALAD

A Perfect and Classic Recipe for Family Breakfast

Easy

25 minutes

Breakfast

4 Servings

INGREDIENTS

1 lb. zucchini, cut into slices

2 tbsp. tomato paste

½ tbsp. tarragon, chopped

1 yellow squash, diced

½ lb. carrots, peeled and diced

1 tbsp. olive oil

Pepper

Salt

COOKING STEPS

1. In an air fryer-baking dish, mix together zucchini, tomato paste, tarragon, squash, carrots, pepper, and salt. Drizzle with olive oil.

2. Place in the air fryer and cook at 400 F for 25 minutes. Stir halfway through.

3. Serve and enjoy.

Nutrition: Calories 79, Fat 3 g, Carbohydrates 11 g, Sugar 5 g, Protein 2 g.

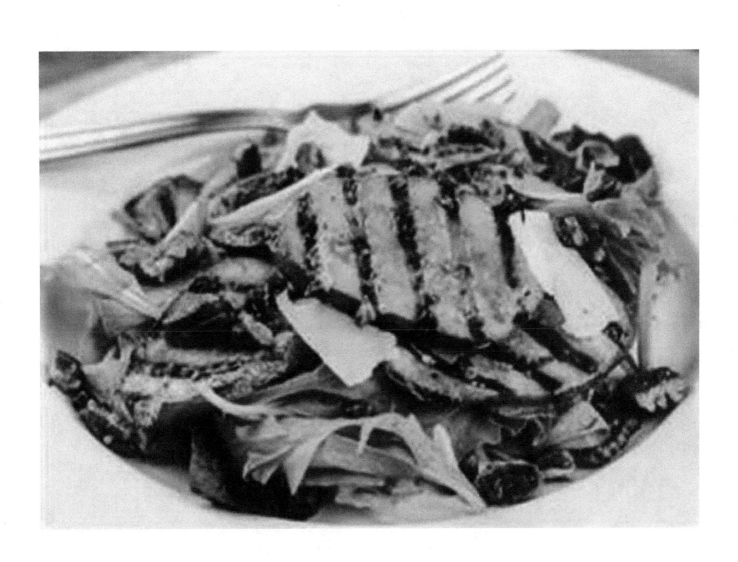

CHAPTER 5: SNACK AND APPETIZERS

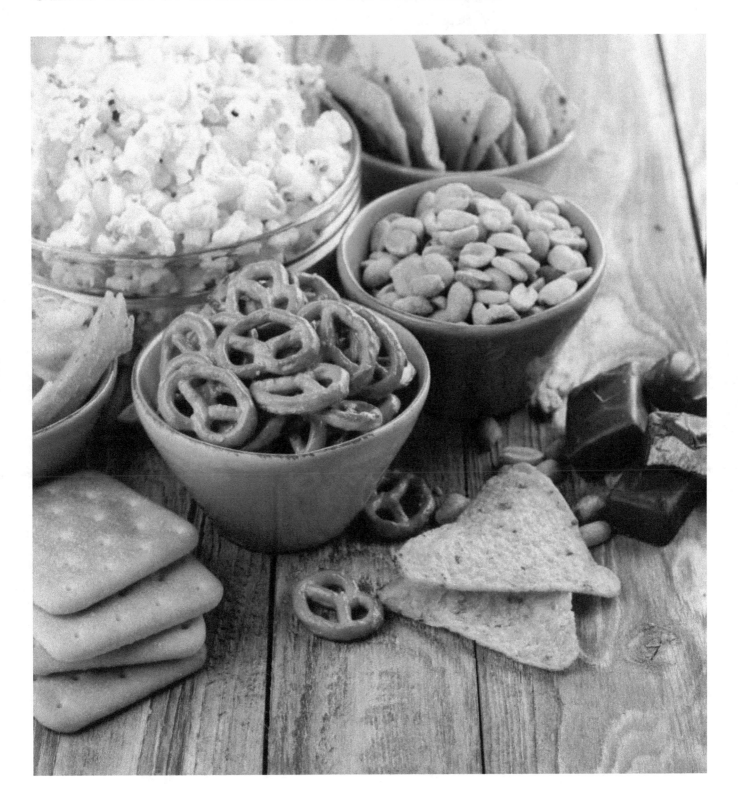

6. CAULIFLOWER POPCORNS

A Perfect Recipe for Snack and Appetizers

| Easy | 12 hours | **Snack and Appetizers** | 4 Servings |

INGREDIENTS

2 pounds head cauliflower, cut into small florets

2 tablespoons hot sauce

1 tablespoon fresh lime juice

1 tablespoon oil

1 tablespoon smoked paprika

1 teaspoon ground cumin

COOKING STEPS

1. In a bowl, add all the ingredients and toss to coat well.

2. Arrange the cauliflower florets onto two cooking trays.

3. Arrange the drip pan at the bottom of the Instant Vortex plus Air Fryer Oven cooking chamber.

4. Select "Dehydrate" and then adjust the temperature to 130 degrees F.

5. Set the timer for 12 hours and press the "Start".

6. When the display shows, "Add Food" insert one tray in the top position and another in the bottom position.

7. When the display shows "Turn Food" do not turn the food but switch the position of cooking trays.

8. When cooking time is complete, remove the trays from Vortex and serve hot.

Nutrition: Calories 95, Fat 4g, Carbohydrates 13.4 g, Sugar 5.7, Protein 4.9 g.

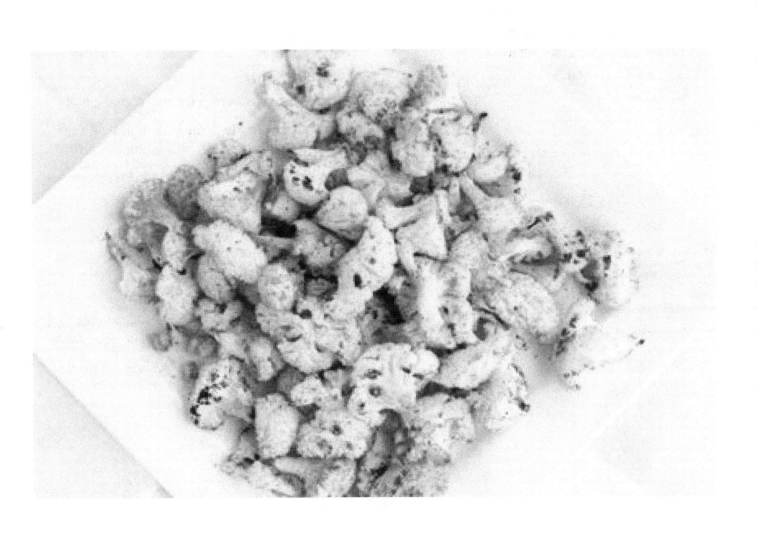

7. KALE CHIPS

A Perfect Recipe for Snack and Appetizers

| Easy | 7 minutes | **Snack and Appetizers** | 4 Servings |

INGREDIENTS

1 (8-ounce) bunch curly kale, tough ribs removed and torn into 2-inch pieces

1 tablespoon olive oil

1 teaspoon salt

COOKING STEPS

1. In a large bowl, add all the ingredients and with your hands, massage the oil and salt into kale completely.

2. Arrange the kale pieces onto two cooking trays.

3. Arrange the drip pan at the bottom of the Instant Vortex plus Air Fryer Oven cooking chamber.

4. Select "Air Dry" and then adjust the temperature to 340 degrees F.

5. Set the timer for 7 minutes and press the "Start".

6. When the display shows, "Add Food" insert one tray in the top position and another in the bottom position.

7. When the display shows "Turn Food" do not turn the food but switch the position of cooking trays.

8. When cooking time is complete, remove the trays from Vortex and transfer the kale chips into a bowl.

Nutrition: Calories 58, Fat 3.5g, Carbohydrates 5.9 g, Sugar 0, Protein 1.7 g.

8. POTATO FRIES

A Perfect Recipe for Snack and Appetizers

 Easy   16 minutes   **Snack and Appetizers**   2 Servings

INGREDIENTS

½ pound potatoes, peeled and cut into ½-inch thick sticks lengthwise

1 tablespoon olive oil

Salt and ground black pepper, as required

COOKING STEPS

1. In a large bowl, add all the ingredients and toss to coat well.

2. Arrange the potato sticks onto a cooking tray.

3. Arrange the drip pan at the bottom of the Instant Vortex plus Air Fryer Oven cooking chamber.

4. Select "Air Dry" and then adjust the temperature to 400 degrees F.

5. Set the timer for 16 minutes and press the "Start".

6. When the display shows, "Add Food" insert the cooking tray in the center position.

7. When the display shows, "Turn Food" turn the potato sticks.

8. When cooking time is complete, remove the tray from Vortex and serve warm.

Nutrition: Calories 138, Fat 7.1g, Carbohydrates 17.8 g, Sugar 1.3, Protein 1.9 g.

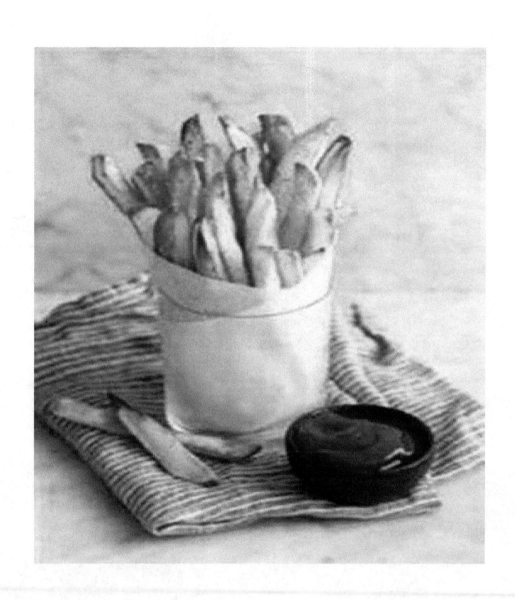

9. ONION RINGS

A Perfect Recipe for Snack and Appetizers

Easy

8 minutes

Snack and Appetizers

4 Servings

INGREDIENTS

1 large onion, cut into ½-inch thick rings

3 tablespoons coconut flour

Salt, as required

2 large eggs

2/3 cup pork rinds

3 tablespoons blanched almond flour

½ teaspoon paprika

½ teaspoon garlic powder

COOKING STEPS

1. In a shallow dish, mix the coconut flour and salt.

2. In a second shallow dish, add the eggs and beat lightly.

3. In a third shallow dish, mix the pork rinds, almond flour, and spices.

4. Coat the onion rings with flour mixture, then dip into egg whites and finally coat with the pork rind mixture.

5. Arrange the coated onion rings onto two lightly greased cooking trays in a single layer.

6. Arrange the drip pan at the bottom of the Instant Vortex plus Air Fryer Oven cooking chamber.

7. Select "Air Dry" and then adjust the temperature to 400 degrees F.

8. Set the timer for 8 minutes and press the "Start".

9. When the display shows, "Add Food" insert one tray in the top position and another in the bottom position.

10. When the display shows "Turn Food" do not turn the food but switch the position of cooking trays.

11. When cooking time is complete, remove the trays from Vortex and serve hot.

Nutrition: Calories 180, Fat 10.2g, Carbohydrates 9 g, Sugar 1.9, Protein 13.7 g.

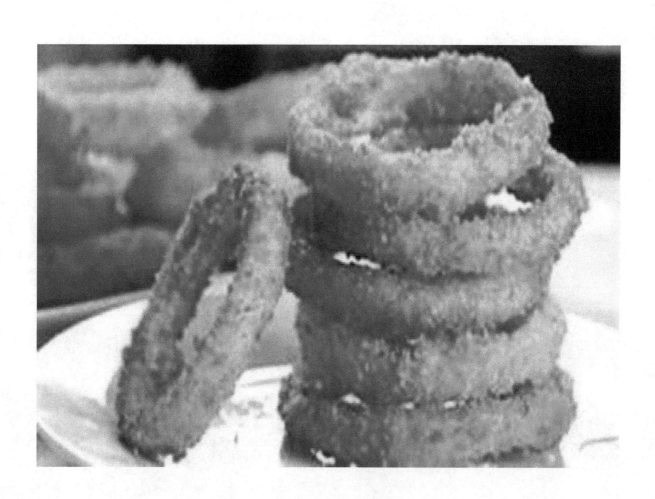

10. CRISPY PICKLE SLICES

A Perfect Recipe for Snack and Appetizers

Easy

18 minutes

Snack and Appetizers

8 Servings

INGREDIENTS

16 dill pickle slices

¼ cup all-purpose flour

Salt, as required

2 small eggs, beaten lightly

1 tablespoon dill pickle juice

¼ teaspoon garlic powder

¼ teaspoon cayenne pepper

1 cup panko breadcrumbs

1 tablespoon fresh dill, minced

Cooking spray

COOKING STEPS

1. Place the pickle slices over paper towels for about 15 minutes or until all the liquid is absorbed.

2. Meanwhile, in a shallow dish, mix the flour and salt.

3. In another shallow dish, add the eggs, pickle juice, garlic powder, and cayenne and beat until well combined.

4. In a third shallow dish, mix the panko and dill.

5. Coat the pickle slices with flour mixture, then dip into the egg mixture and finally coat with the panko mixture.

6. Spray the pickle slices with cooking spray.

7. Arrange the pickle slice onto a cooking tray.

8. Arrange the drip pan at the bottom of the Instant Vortex plus Air Fryer Oven cooking chamber.

9. Select "Air Dry" and then adjust the temperature to 400 degrees F.

10. Set the timer for 18 minutes and press the "Start".

11. When the display shows, "Add Food" insert the cooking tray in the center position.

12. When the display shows, "Turn Food" turn the pickle slices.

13. When cooking time is complete, remove the tray from Vortex and serve warm.

Nutrition: Calories 80, Fat 2g, Carbohydrates 6 g, Sugar 0.3, Protein 2.1 g.

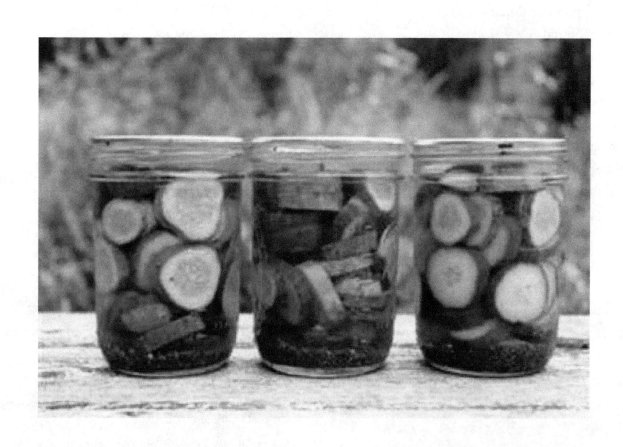

11. BEEF TAQUITOS

A Perfect Recipe for Snack and Appetizers

 Easy
 8 minutes
 Snack and Appetizers
 6 Servings

INGREDIENTS

6 corn tortillas
2 cups cooked beef, shredded
½ cup onion, chopped
1 cup pepper jack cheese, shredded
Olive oil cooking spray

COOKING STEPS

1. Arrange the tortillas onto a smooth surface.

2. Place the shredded meat over one corner of each tortilla, followed by onion and cheese.

3. Roll each tortilla to secure the filling and secure with toothpicks.

4. Spray each taquito with cooking spray evenly.

5. Arrange the taquitos onto a cooking tray.

6. Arrange the drip pan at the bottom of the Instant Vortex plus Air Fryer Oven cooking chamber.

7. Select "Air Dry" and then adjust the temperature to 400 degrees F.

8. Set the timer for 8 minutes and press the "Start".

9. When the display shows, "Add Food" insert the cooking tray in the center position.

10. When the display shows, "Turn Food" turn the taquitos.

11. When cooking time is complete, remove the tray from Vortex and serve warm.

Nutrition: Calories 263, Fat 10.7g, Carbohydrates 12.3 g, Sugar 0.6, Protein 28.4 g.

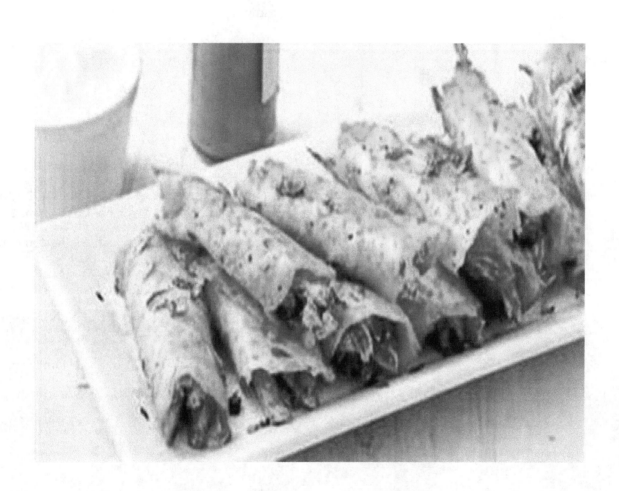

12. CHEESE SANDWICH

A Perfect Recipe for Snack and Appetizers

| Easy | 10 minutes | **Snack and Appetizers** | 2 Servings |

INGREDIENTS

3 tablespoons butter, softened

4 white bread slices

2 cheddar cheese slices

COOKING STEPS

1. Spread the butter over each bread slice generously.

2. Place 2 bread slices onto a cooking tray, buttered side down

3. Top each buttered bread slice with one cheese slice.

4. Cover with the remaining bread slices, buttered side up.

5. Arrange the sandwiches onto a cooking tray.

6. Arrange the drip pan at the bottom of the Instant Vortex plus Air Fryer Oven cooking chamber.

7. Select "Air Dry" and then adjust the temperature to 375 degrees F.

8. Set the timer for 10 minutes and press the "Start".

9. When the display shows, "Add Food" insert the cooking tray in the center position.

10. When the display shows, "Turn Food" turn the sandwiches.

11. When cooking time is complete, remove the tray from Vortex.

12. Cut each sandwich in half vertically and serve warm.

Nutrition: Calories 307, Fat 27.2g, Carbohydrates 9.4 g, Sugar 0.8, Protein 8.4 g.

13. AIR FRYER APPLE SLICES
A Perfect Recipe for Snack and Appetizers

Easy

10 minutes

Snack and Appetizers

1 Servings

INGREDIENTS

1 apple, core and slice ¼-inch thick

¼ tsp ground cinnamon

Pinch of salt

COOKING STEPS

1. Spray air fryer oven tray with cooking spray.

2. Arrange apple slices on the tray and sprinkle them with cinnamon and salt.

3. Air fry at 390 F for 10-12 minutes. Turn apple slices halfway through.

4. Serve and enjoy.

Nutrition: Calories 52, Fat 0g, Carbohydrates 13.8 g, Sugar 10.4, Protein 0.3 g.

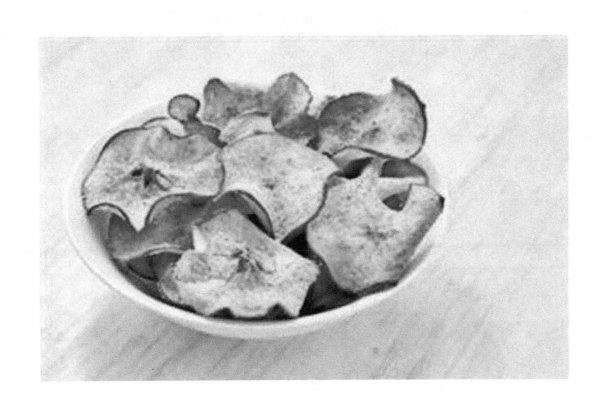

14. SIMPLE POTATO CHIPS

A Perfect Recipe for Snack and Appetizers

Easy

9 minutes

Snack and Appetizers

1 Servings

INGREDIENTS

2 potatoes, scrubbed and washed
2 tbsp. olive oil
Pepper
Salt

COOKING STEPS

1. Slice potatoes 1-inch thick slices using a mandolin slicer.

2. Add potato slices into the mixing bowl. Add oil, pepper, and salt to the bowl and toss until potato slices are well coated.

3. Arrange potato slices on an air fryer oven tray and cook at 370 F for 3 minutes.

4. Turn potato slices to the other side and air fry for 3 minutes more.

5. Again, turn potato slices and air fry for 3 minutes more.

6. Serve and enjoy.

Nutrition: Calories 293, Fat 14.5g, Carbohydrates 36.6 g, Sugar 1.7, Protein 4.1 g.

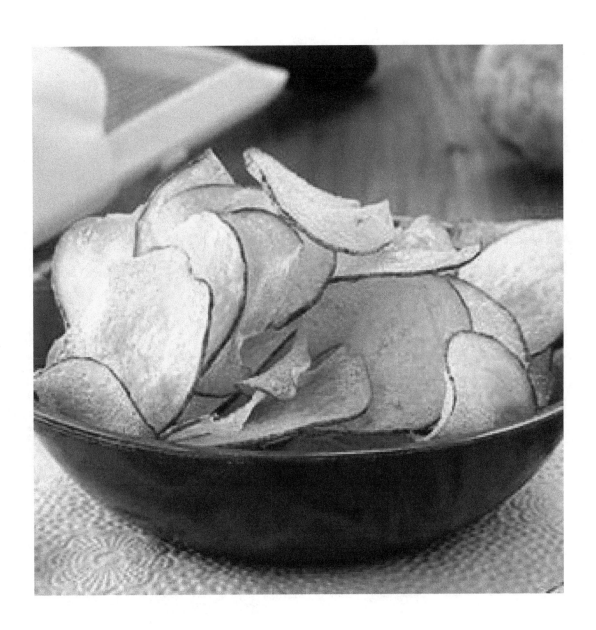

CHAPTER 6: VEGETABLE RECIPES

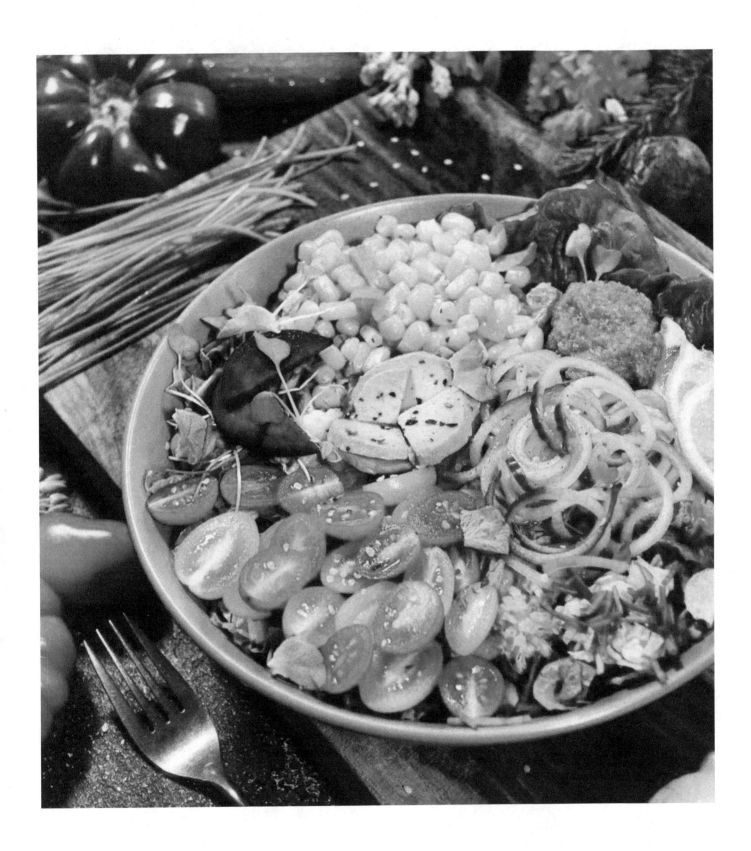

15. AIR FRYER POTATO CHIPS

A Perfect Recipe for Vegetable

Easy   15 minutes   **vegetable recipes**   4 Servings

INGREDIENTS

1 large Russet Potato

Grapeseed Oil Cooking Spray

Sea Salt

COOKING STEPS

1. Use a paper towel to press out as much of the moisture from the potatoes slices as possible. Now spray the basket of your air fryer toaster oven with the oil spray and put the potatoes in a single layer inside. You will have to do this in batches. Spray the tops of the potatoes with the oil spray and sprinkle with salt. Turn your air fryer to 450 degrees F and cook until the corners of the potatoes are golden brown and crisp depending on how thin your potatoes are. Take out the chips from the air fryer and let them crisp up on the counter overnight.

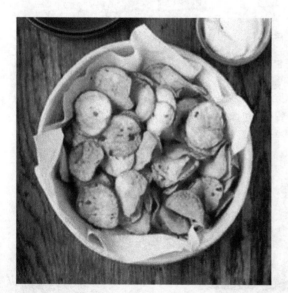

Nutrition: Calories 75, Fat 1 g, Carbohydrates 18 g, Protein 2 g.

16. AIR FRYER SUSHI ROLLS

A Perfect Recipe for Vegetable

Easy

15 minutes

vegetable recipes

3 Servings

INGREDIENTS

1/2 cups chopped kale

3/4 tsp. toasted sesame oil

1/2 tsp. rice vinegar

1/8 tsp. garlic powder

1/4 tsp. ground ginger

3/4 tsp. soy sauce

1 tbsp. sesame seeds

3 sheets of sushi nori

1/2 of a Haas avocado

Sriracha sauce to taste

1/2 cup panko breadcrumbs

1/4 cup vegan mayonnaise

1 batch Pressure Cooker Sushi Rice

COOKING STEPS

1. Add the kale, vinegar, sesame oil, garlic powder, ground ginger, and soy sauce in a bowl. Massage the kale until it turns bright green and wilted. Mix in the sesame seeds, and set aside. Make sushi rolls lay out a sheet of nori on a dry surface. Grab a handful of rice, and spread it onto the nori. The idea here is to get a thin layer of rice covering almost the entire sheet. Along one edge, you will want to leave about 1/2" of naked seaweed. On the end of the seaweed opposite that naked part, a layout about 2-3 tablespoons of kale salad, and top with a couple of slices of avocado. Make sushi rolls by starting from the filled side. When you get to the end, use that naked bit of seaweed to seal the roll closed. Get your fingertips wet, and moisten that bit of seaweed to make it stick. Carry on with steps to make 3 more sushi rolls. Make the Sriracha Mayo. In a shallow bowl, whisk together the vegan mayo with sriracha, until you reach the heat level that you like. Start with 1 tsp. add more, 1/2 teaspoon at a time, until you have the spicy mayo. Pour the panko breadcrumbs into a shallow bowl. Take the sushi roll, and coat it as evenly as possible in the Sriracha Mayo, then in the panko. Place the roll into your air fryer toaster oven basket. Repeat with the rest of your sushi rolls. Use air fryer to fry at 390 degrees F for 10 minutes, shaking gently after 5 minutes. When the rolls are cool enough to handle, grab a good knife, and very gently slice the roll into 6-8 pieces. When you're slicing, think of gently sawing, and don't press hard with your knife. That will just send kale and avocado flying out of the ends of your roll. Serve with soy sauce for dipping.

Nutrition: Calories 470, Fat 22 g, Carbohydrates 50 g, Protein 18 g.

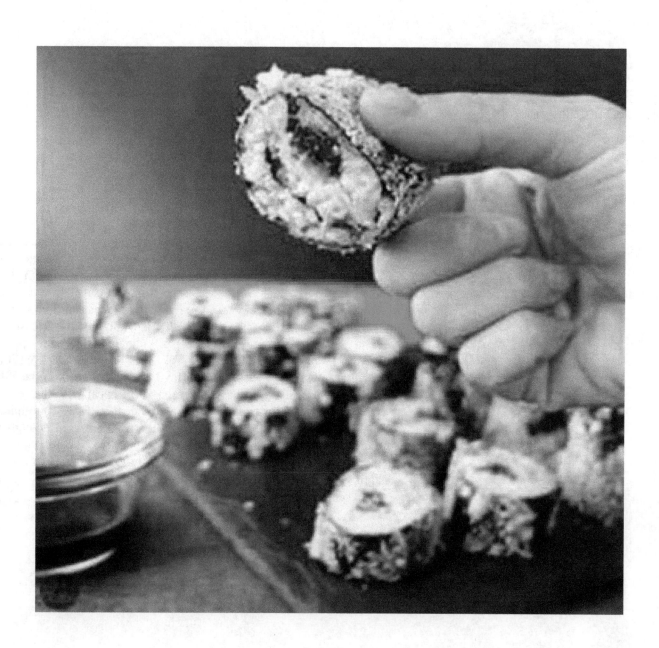

17. CHICKPEA CAULIFLOWER TACOS

A Perfect Recipe for Vegetable

Easy

30 minutes

vegetable recipes

4 Servings

INGREDIENTS

4 cups cauliflower

2 tbsp. olive oil

2 tbsp. taco seasoning

8 small tortillas

2 avocados sliced

19 oz. rinsed chickpeas

4 cups cabbage shredded

Coconut yogurt to drizzle

COOKING STEPS

1. Preheat of air fryer toaster oven to 390 degrees F. Toss the cauliflower and chickpeas with the olive oil and taco seasoning in a bowl. Place everything into the basket of your air fryer. Shaking the basket occasionally for 20 minutes or until cooked through. Serve the tacos with avocado slices, cabbage, and coconut yogurt.

Nutrition: Calories 395, Fat 14 g, Carbohydrates 58 g, Protein 13 g.

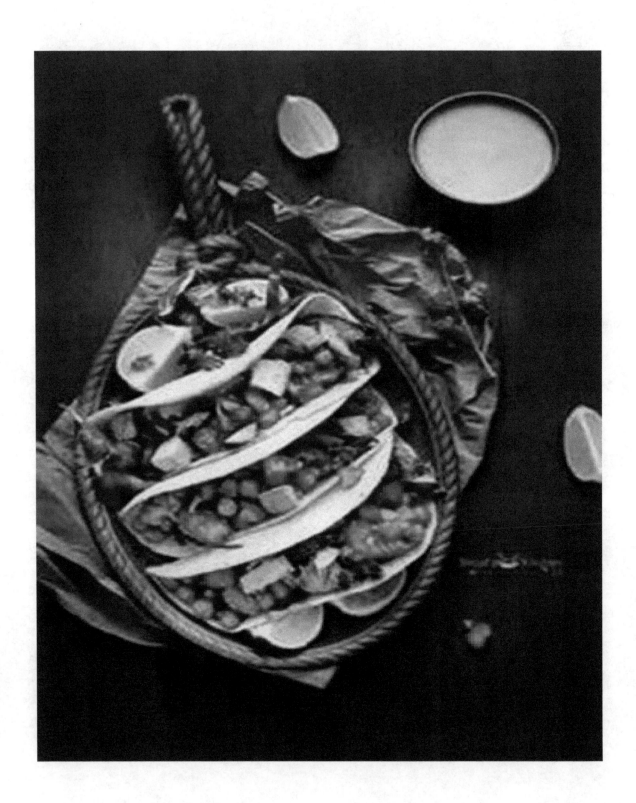

18. KALE AND POTATO NUGGETS

A Perfect Recipe for Vegetable

Easy

25 minutes

vegetable recipes

4 Servings

INGREDIENTS

2 cups chopped potatoes

4 cups chopped kale

1 tsp. olive oil

1 clove garlic minced

1/8 cup almond milk

1/4 teaspoon sea salt

1/8 tsp. black pepper

Vegetable oil spray as needed

COOKING STEPS

1. Place the potatoes in a large pan of boiling water. Cook for about 30 minutes. In a skillet, heat the oil over medium to high heat. Add the garlic and sauté until it becomes golden brown. Put the kale and sauté for 2 to 3 minutes. Shift to a large bowl. Transfer the cooked potatoes to a medium bowl. Add the salt, milk, pepper, and mash with a fork. Shift the potatoes to the large bowl and combine with the cooked kale. Preheat the air fryer toaster oven to 390°F for 5 minutes. Roll down the potato and kale mixture into 1-inch nuggets. Spray the air fryer basket with vegetable oil. Put the nuggets in the air fryer and cook for 12 to 15 minutes, until golden brown, shaking at 6 minutes.

Nutrition: Calories 355, Fat 14 g, Carbohydrates 45 g, Protein 13 g.

19. AIR FRYER LEMON TOFU

A Perfect Recipe for Vegetable

 Easy

 25 minutes

 vegetable recipes

 4 Servings

INGREDIENTS

1 lb. firm tofu

2 tbsp. organic sugar

1 tbsp. tamari

1 tsp. lemon zest

1/2 cup water

1/3 cup lemon juice

3 tbsp. cornstarch or arrowroot powder

COOKING STEPS

1. Slice the tofu into cubes. Put the tofu cubes in a storage bag. Seal the bag after adding the tamari. Shake the bag so that all the tofu is coated with the tamari. Add the tbsp. of cornstarch to the bag. Shake again so that the tofu is coated. Place the tofu aside to marinate for at least 15 minutes. During the time add all the sauce ingredients to a small bowl and mix with a spoon. Put the tofu in the air fryer toaster oven in a single layer. Now cook the tofu at 390 degrees for 10 minutes, shaking it after 5 minutes. When you're done cooking the batches of tofu, place it all in a skillet over medium to high heat. Mix the sauce and pour it over the tofu. Mix the tofu and sauce until the sauce has thickened and the tofu is heated through too.

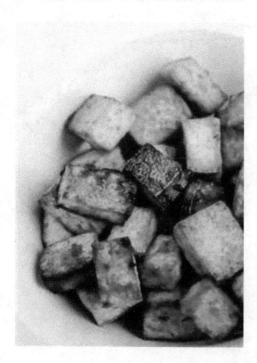

Nutrition: Calories 355, Fat 14 g, Carbohydrates 45 g, Protein 13 g.

20. AIR FRYER CLASSY FALAFEL

A Perfect Recipe for Vegetable

Easy

45 minutes

vegetable recipes

8 Servings

INGREDIENTS

1/2 cup dry garbanzo beans

7 cloves garlic

1/2 cup chopped fresh parsley

2 tbsp. flour

1/2 cup chopped fresh cilantro

1/2 tsp. sea salt

1/2 cup chopped white onion

1/8 tsp. ground cardamom

1 tsp. ground coriander

COOKING STEPS

1. Overnight soak: Put dried garbanzo beans in a large bowl and cover with 1 inch of water. Left it uncovered for 20-24 hours. Drain completely. Quick soak: Rinse garbanzo beans and add to a large pot. Cover them with 2 inches of water and bring to a boil. Let it boil for 1 minute, cover the pot, and remove from heat. Let it stand for 1 hour. Drain completely. In the food processor's bowl add parsley, cilantro, onion, and garlic. Mix until well combined. Put soaked garbanzo beans, flour, salt, cumin, cardamom, coriander, and cayenne in a food processor. Grind until ingredients form a rough, coarse meal. Put mixture into a bowl, cover, and refrigerate it for 1-2 hours to allow flavors to come together. Once it is cooled, remove it from the refrigerator and form into 1½-inch balls, then form patties. Preheat of air fryer toaster oven to 400 degrees F. Spray the fryer basket with oil. Put falafel into a basket. Now cook for 10 minutes. Do the same with the remaining falafel.

Nutrition: Calories 150, Fat 2.5 g, Carbohydrates 25 g, Protein 8 g.

21. AIR FRYER THAI VEGETARIAN BITE

A Perfect Recipe for Vegetable

| Easy | 25 minutes | **vegetable recipes** | 16 Servings |

INGREDIENTS

1 Broccoli

Salt & Pepper

1 Cauliflower

1 Tsp Cumin

6 Carrots

1 tbsp. Mixed Spice

1/2 cauliflower

1 tbsp. Coriander

1 Courgette

2 Leeks

50g Plain Flour

1 tbsp. Olive Oil

1 Onion peeled

1 cm Cube Ginger

1 tbsp. Garlic Puree

1 Can Coconut Milk

1 tbsp. Thai Green Curry Paste

Handful Garden Peas

COOKING STEPS

1. Cook your onion in a wok with garlic, ginger, and olive oil until the onion has a good bit of color on it. When you are cooking your onion in a steamer cook your vegetables (apart from the courgette and leek) for 20 minutes or until they are nearly cooked. Put the courgette, the leek, and the curry paste into your wok and cook on medium heat for a more 5 minutes. Put the coconut milk and the rest of the seasoning mix well and then add the cauliflower rice. Mix them again and allow it to simmer for 10 minutes. Add the steamed vegetables once it has simmered for 10 minutes and the sauce has reduced by half. Stir well and you will now have a lovely base for your veggie bites. Put in the fridge for an hour to allow it to cool. After one hour makes it into bite sizes and place in the air fryer toaster oven. Now Cook for 10 minutes at 180C and then eat with a cooling dip.

Nutrition: Calories 117, Fat 7 g, Carbohydrates 12 g, Protein 2 g.

22. GARLIC AND HERB ROASTED CHICKPEAS

A Perfect Recipe for Vegetable

 Easy

 25 minutes

 vegetable recipes

 4 Servings

INGREDIENTS

2 can of chickpeas

1 tbsp. nutritional yeast

1 tbsp. olive oil

2 tsp garlic powder

1 tbsp. mixed herbs

Sea salt and black pepper

COOKING STEPS

1. Drain the chickpeas and then add to a medium-sized mixing bowl and add in the olive oil and seasonings. Mix them well to combine using a spatula, ensuring all chickpeas are well coated. Distribute and cook in two batches in the air fryer toaster oven at 200°C for 15-20 minutes and stirring once every 10 minutes. Once they were done they were golden brown and crispy all the way through. Eat while warm and store in an airtight jar once cooled to preserve crispiness.

Nutrition: Calories 395, Fat 14 g, Carbohydrates 58 g, Protein 13 g.

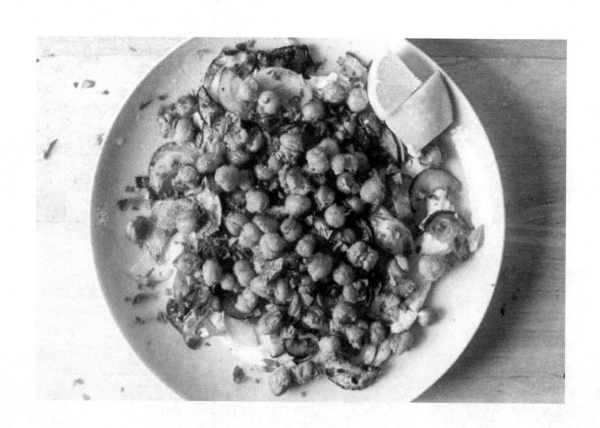

CHAPTER 7: POULTRY RECIPES

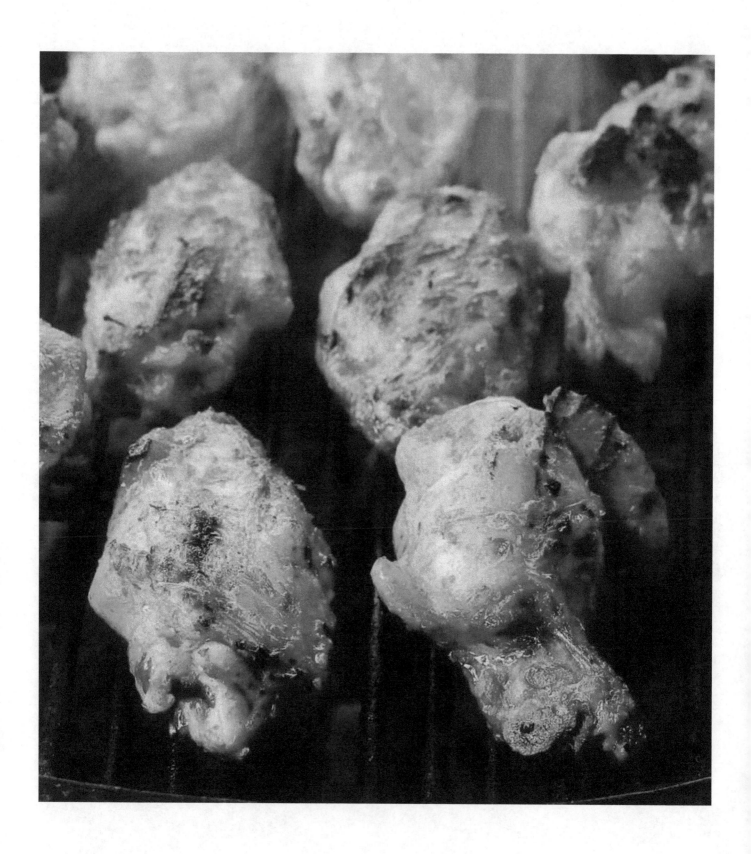

23. BUFFALO CHICKEN WINGS

A Perfect Classic Recipe for Poultry

Easy

30 minutes

Poultry Recipes

8 Servings

INGREDIENTS

1 tsp. salt

1-2 tbsp. brown sugar

1 tbsp. Worcestershire sauce

½ C. vegan butter

½ C. cayenne pepper sauce

4 pounds of chicken wings

COOKING STEPS

1. Whisk salt, brown sugar, Worcestershire sauce, butter, and hot sauce together and set to the side.

2. Dry wings and add to the air fryer basket.

3. Set temperature to 380°F, and set time to 25 minutes. Cook tossing halfway through.

4. When the timer sounds, shake wings and bump up the temperature to 400 degrees and cook for another 5 minutes.

5. Take out wings and place them into a big bowl. Add sauce and toss well.

6. Serve alongside celery sticks.

Nutrition: Calories 402 g, Fat 16 g, Carbohydrates 37 g, Protein 17 g

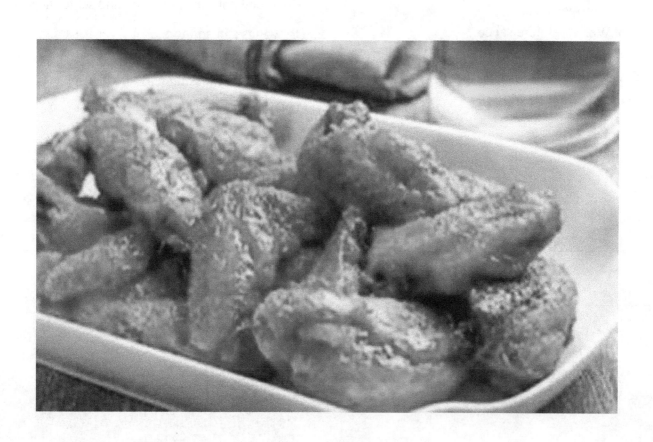

24. ZINGY & NUTTY CHICKEN WINGS

A Perfect Classic Recipe for Poultry

Easy   18 minutes   **Poultry Recipes**   4 Servings

INGREDIENTS

1 tablespoon fish sauce

1 tablespoon fresh lemon juice

1 teaspoon sugar

12 chicken middle wings, cut into half

2 fresh lemongrass stalks, chopped finely

¼ cup unsalted cashews, crushed

COOKING STEPS

1. In a bowl, mix fish sauce, lime juice, and sugar.

2. Add wings ad coat with mixture generously. Refrigerate to marinate for about 1-2 hours.

3. Preheat the air fryer oven to 355 degrees F.

4. In the air fryer oven pan, place lemongrass stalks. Cook for about 2-3 minutes. Remove the cashew mixture from Air fryer and transfer it into a bowl. Now, set the air fryer oven to 390 degrees F.

5. Place the chicken wings in the air fryer pan. Cook for about 13-15 minutes further.

6. Transfer the wings into serving plates. Sprinkle with cashew mixture and serve.

Nutrition: Calories 81 g, Fat 5.4 g, Carbohydrates 0 g, Protein 7.4 g

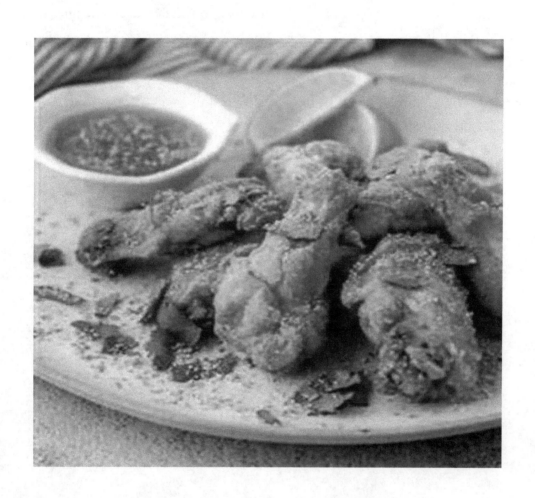

25. HONEY AND WINE CHICKEN BREASTS

A Perfect Classic Recipe for Poultry

 Easy

 15 minutes

 Poultry Recipes

 4 Servings

INGREDIENTS

2 chicken breasts, rinsed and halved

1 tablespoon melted butter

1/2 teaspoon freshly ground pepper, or to taste

3/4 teaspoon sea salt, or to taste

1 teaspoon paprika

1 teaspoon dried rosemary

2 tablespoons dry white wine

1 tablespoon honey

COOKING STEPS

1. Firstly, pat the chicken breasts dry. Lightly coat them with the melted butter.

2. Then, add the remaining ingredients.

3. Transfer them to the air fryer basket; bake for about 15 minutes at 330 degrees F. Serve warm and enjoy!

Nutrition: Calories 189 g, Fat 14 g, sugar 1 g, Protein 11 g

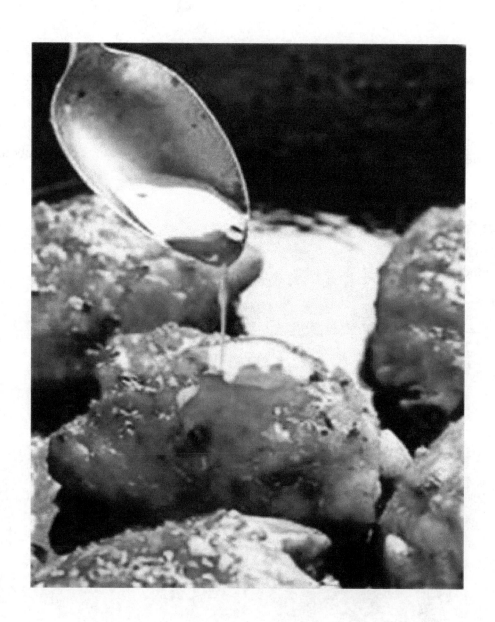

26. CHICKEN FILLETS, BRIE & HAM

A Perfect Classic Recipe for Poultry

Easy

15 minutes

Poultry Recipes

4 Servings

INGREDIENTS

2 Large Chicken Fillets

Freshly Ground Black Pepper

4 Small Slices of Brie (Or your cheese of choice)

1 Tbsp. Freshly Chopped Chives

4 Slices Cured Ham

COOKING STEPS

1. Slice the fillets into four and make incisions as you would for a hamburger bun. Leave a little "hinge" uncut at the back. Season the inside and pop some brie and chives in there. Close them, and wrap them each in a slice of ham. Brush with oil and pop them into the basket.

2. Heat your fryer to 350° F. Pour into the Oven rack/basket. Place the Rack on the middle-shelf of the Air fryer oven. Set temperature to 400°F, and set time to 15 minutes. Roast the little parcels until they look tasty (15 min)

Nutrition: Calories 216.4 g, Fat 6.4 g, Carbohydrates 10.9 g, Protein 27.2 g, Sugar 0.9.

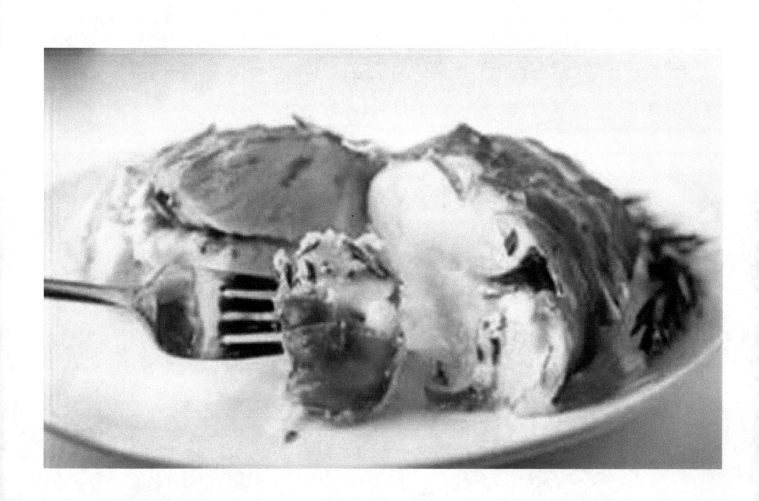

27. CHICKEN FAJITAS

A Perfect Classic Recipe for Poultry

| Easy | 10 minutes | **Poultry Recipes** | 4 Servings |

INGREDIENTS

4 boneless, skinless chicken breasts, sliced

1 small red onion, sliced

2 red bell peppers, sliced

½ cup spicy ranch salad dressing, divided

½ teaspoon dried oregano

8 corn tortillas

2 cups torn butter lettuce

2 avocados, peeled and chopped

COOKING STEPS

1. Place the chicken, onion, and pepper in the air fryer basket. Drizzle with 1 tablespoon of the salad dressing and add the oregano. Toss to combine.

2. Place the Rack on the middle-shelf of the Air fryer oven. Set temperature to 165°F, and set time to 14 minutes. Grill for 10 to 14 minutes or until the chicken is 165°F on a food thermometer. Transfer the chicken and vegetables to a bowl and toss with the remaining salad dressing. Serve the chicken mixture with the tortillas, lettuce, and avocados and let everyone make their creations.

Nutrition: Calories 783 g, Fat 38 g, Fiber 12 g, Protein 72 g.

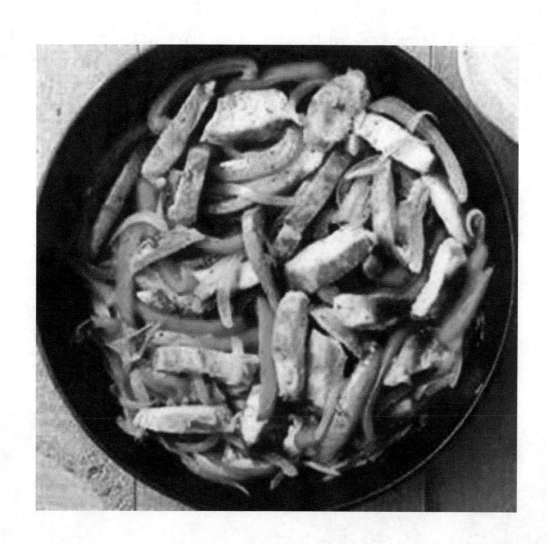

28. CRISPY HONEY GARLIC CHICKEN WINGS

A Perfect Classic Recipe for Poultry

 Easy

 25 minutes

 Poultry Recipes

 8 Servings

INGREDIENTS

1/8 C. water

½ tsp. salt

4 tbsp. minced garlic

¼ C. vegan butter

¼ C. raw honey

¾ C. almond flour

16 chicken wings

COOKING STEPS

1. Rinse off and dry chicken wings well.

2. Spray air fryer basket with olive oil.

3. Coat chicken wings with almond flour and add coated wings to the air fryer.

4. Pour into the Oven basket. Place the basket on the middle shelf of the Air fryer oven. Set temperature to 380°F, and set time to 25 minutes. Cook shaking every 5 minutes.

5. When the timer goes off, cook 5-10 minutes at 400 degrees until the skin becomes crispy and dry.

6. As chicken cooks, melt butter in a saucepan and add garlic. Sauté garlic 5 minutes. Add salt and honey, simmer 20 minutes. Make sure to stir every so often, so the sauce does not burn. Add a bit of water after 15 minutes to ensure the sauce does not harden.

7. Take out chicken wings from the air fryer and coat in sauce. Enjoy!

Nutrition: Calories 435 g, Fat 19 g, Protein 31 g, Sugar 6.

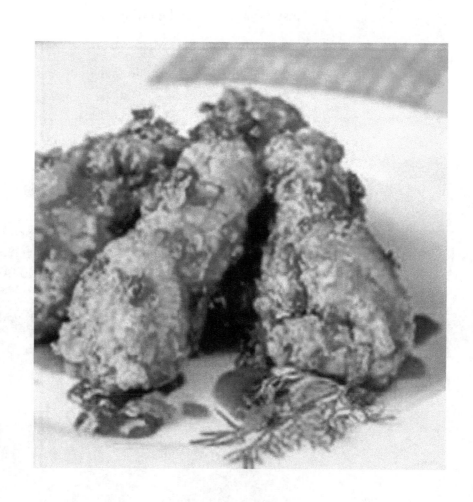

29. BBQ CHICKEN RECIPE FROM GREECE

A Perfect Classic Recipe for Poultry

Easy

25 minutes

Poultry Recipes

4 Servings

INGREDIENTS

1 (8 ounces) container fat-free plain yogurt

2 tablespoons fresh lemon juice

2 teaspoons dried oregano

1-pound skinless, boneless chicken breast halves - cut into 1-inch pieces

1 large red onion, cut into wedges

1/2 teaspoon lemon zest

1/2 teaspoon salt

1 large green bell pepper, cut into 1 1/2-inch piece

1/3 cup crumbled feta cheese with basil and sun-dried tomatoes

1/4 teaspoon ground black pepper

1/4 teaspoon crushed dried rosemary

COOKING STEPS

1. Rinse off and dry chicken wings well.

2. Spray air fryer basket with olive oil.

3. Coat chicken wings with almond flour and add coated wings to the air fryer.

4. Pour into the Oven basket. Place the basket on the middle shelf of the Air fryer oven. Set temperature to 380°F, and set time to 25 minutes. Cook shaking every 5 minutes.

5. When the timer goes off, cook 5-10 minutes at 400 degrees until the skin becomes crispy and dry.

6. As chicken cooks, melt butter in a saucepan and add garlic. Sauté garlic 5 minutes. Add salt and honey, simmer 20 minutes. Make sure to stir every so often, so the sauce does not burn. Add a bit of water after 15 minutes to ensure the sauce does not harden.

7. Take out chicken wings from the air fryer and coat in sauce. Enjoy!

Nutrition: Calories 242 g, Fat 7 g, Protein 31 g, Sugar 6.

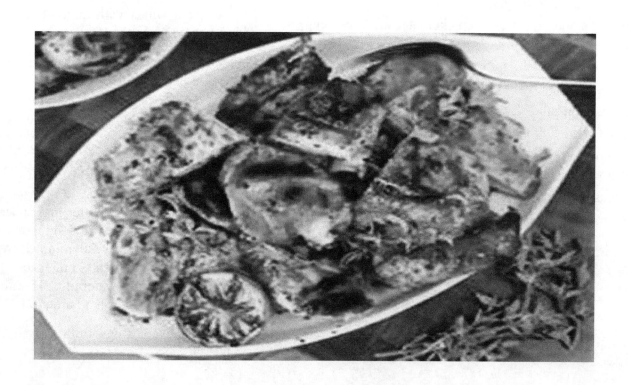

30. CHICKEN-FRIED STEAK SUPREME

A Perfect Classic Recipe for Poultry

| Easy | 30 minutes | **Poultry Recipes** | 8 Servings |

INGREDIENTS

½ pound beef-bottom round, sliced into strips

1 cup of breadcrumbs (Panko brand works well)

2 medium-sized eggs

Pinch of salt and pepper

½ tablespoon of ground thyme

COOKING STEPS

1. Cover the basket of the air fryer oven with a lining of tin foil, leaving the edges uncovered to allow air to circulate through the basket. Preheat the air fryer oven to 350 degrees. In a mixing bowl, beat the eggs until fluffy and until the yolks and whites are fully combined, and set aside. In a separate mixing bowl, combine the breadcrumbs, thyme, salt, and pepper, and set aside. One by one, dip each piece of raw steak into the bowl with dry ingredients, coating all sides; then submerge into the bowl with wet ingredients, then dip again into the dry ingredients. This double coating will ensure an extra-crisp air fry. Lay the coated steak pieces on the foil covering the air-fryer basket, in a single flat layer.

2. Set the air fryer oven timer for 15 minutes. After 15 minutes, the air fryer will turn off and the steak should be mid-way cooked and the breaded coating starting to brown. Using tongs, turn each piece of steak over to ensure a full all-over fry. Reset the air fryer oven to 320 degrees for 15 minutes. After 15 minutes, when the air fryer shuts off, remove the fried steak strips using tongs and set them on a serving plate. Eat as soon as cool enough to handle and enjoy!

Nutrition: Calories 1787 g, Fat 116 g, Carbohydrates 71.9 g, Protein 114 g.

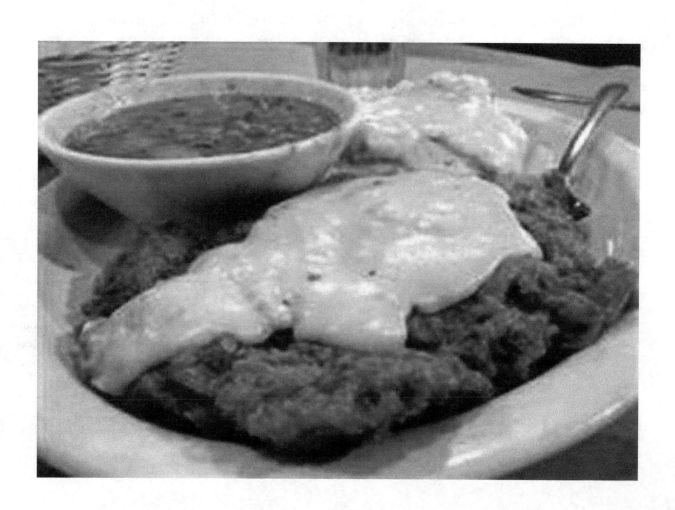

CHAPTER 8: PORK RECIPES

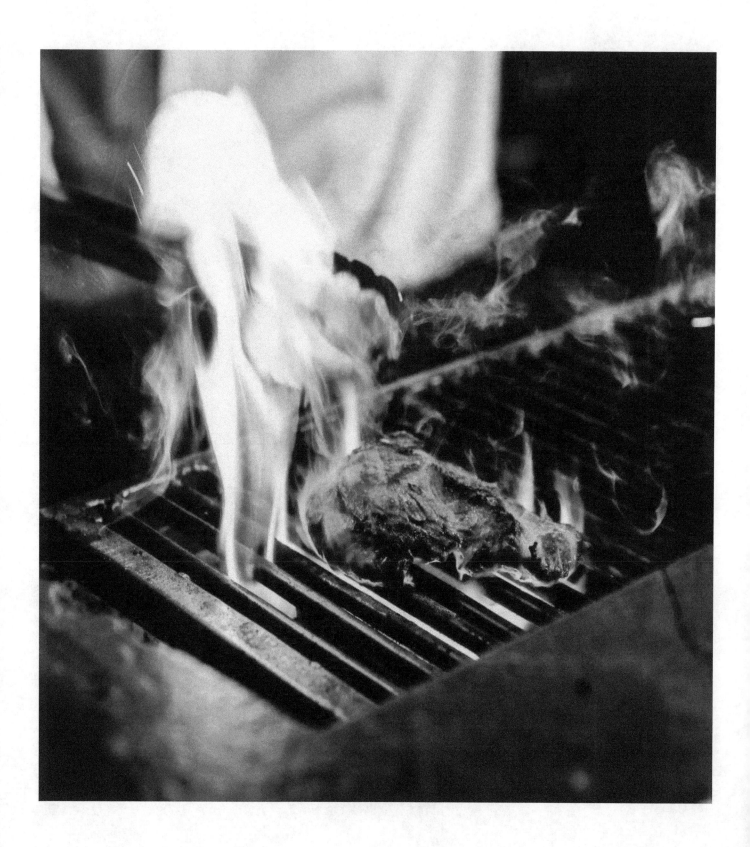

31. CRISPY FRIED PORK CHOPS THE SOUTHERN WAY

A Perfect Classic Recipe for Pork

Easy

25 minutes

Pork Recipes

4 Servings

INGREDIENTS

½ cup all-purpose flour

½ cup low-fat buttermilk

½ teaspoon black pepper

½ teaspoon Tabasco sauce

teaspoon paprika

3 bone-in pork chops

COOKING STEPS

1. Place the buttermilk and hot sauce in a Ziploc bag and add the pork chops. Allow marinating for at least an hour in the fridge.
2. In a bowl, combine the flour, paprika, and black pepper.
3. Remove pork from the Ziploc bag and dredge in the flour mixture.
4. Preheat the air fryer oven to 390°F.
5. Spray the pork chops with cooking oil.
6. Pour into the Oven rack/basket. Place the Rack on the middle-shelf of the Air fryer oven. Set temperature to 390°F, and set time to 25 minutes.

Nutrition: Calories 427, Fat 21 g, Sugar 2 g, Protein 46 g.

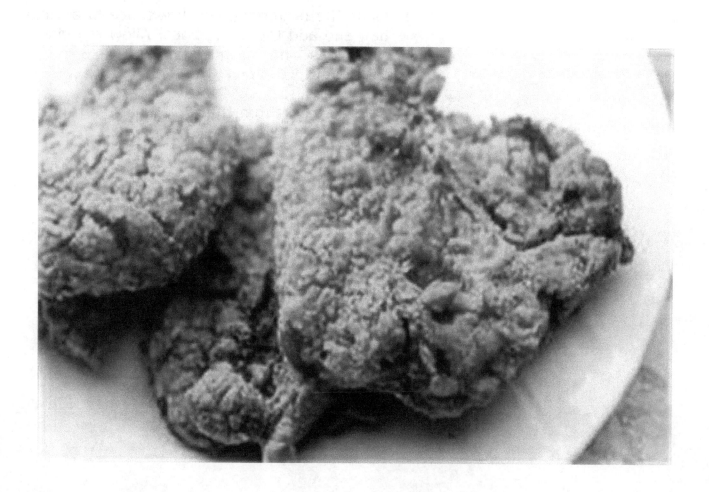

32. FRIED PORK QUESADILLA

A Perfect Classic Recipe for Pork

Easy   12 minutes   **Pork Recipes**   2 Servings

INGREDIENTS

Two 6-inch corn or flour tortilla shells

1 medium-sized pork shoulder, approximately 4 ounces, sliced

½ medium-sized white onion, sliced

½ medium-sized red pepper, sliced

½ medium-sized green pepper, sliced

½ medium-sized yellow pepper, sliced

¼ cup of shredded pepper-jack cheese

¼ cup of shredded mozzarella cheese

COOKING STEPS

1. Preheat the air fryer oven to 350 degrees.

2. In the oven on high heat for 20 minutes, grill the pork, onion, and peppers in foil in the same pan, allowing the moisture from the vegetables and the juice from the pork to mingle together. Remove pork and vegetables in foil from the oven. While they are cooling, sprinkle half the shredded cheese over one of the tortillas, then cover with the pieces of pork, onions, and peppers, and then layer on the rest of the shredded cheese. Top with the second tortilla. Place directly on the hot surface of the air fryer basket.

3. Set the air fryer timer for 6 minutes. After 6 minutes, when the air fryer shuts off, flip the tortillas onto the other side with a spatula, the cheese should be melted enough that it would not fall apart, but be careful anyway not to spill any toppings!

4. Reset the air fryer to 350 degrees for another 6 minutes.

5. After 6 minutes, when the air fryer shuts off, the tortillas should be browned and crisp, and the pork, onion, peppers, and cheese will be crispy, hot, and delicious. Remove with tongs and let sit on a serving plate to cool for a few minutes before slicing.

Nutrition: Calories 122, Fat 3 g, Carbohydrates 0 g, Protein 22 g.

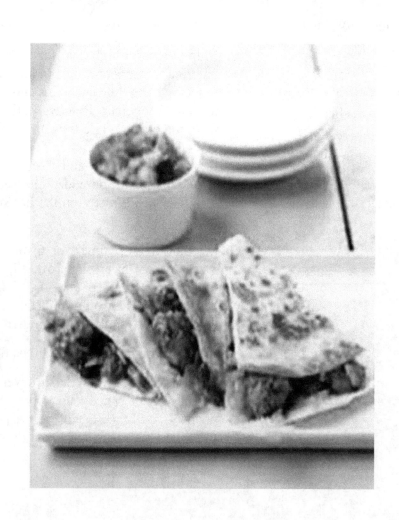

33. PORK WONTON WONDERFUL

A Perfect Classic Recipe for Pork

Easy

25 minutes

Pork Recipes

3 Servings

INGREDIENTS

8 wonton wrappers (Leasa brand works great, though any will do)

4 ounces of raw minced pork

1 medium-sized green apple

1 cup of water, for wetting the wonton wrappers

1 tablespoon of vegetable oil

½ tablespoon of oyster sauce

1 tablespoon of soy sauce

Large pinch of ground white pepper

COOKING STEPS

1. Cover the basket of the air fryer oven with a lining of tin foil, leaving the edges uncovered to allow air to circulate through the basket. Preheat the air fryer to 350 degrees.

2. In a small mixing bowl, combine the oyster sauce, soy sauce, and white pepper, then add in the minced pork and stir thoroughly. Cover and set in the fridge to marinate for at least 15 minutes. Core the apple, and slice into small cubes – smaller than bite-sized chunks.

3. Add the apples to the marinating meat mixture, and combine thoroughly. Spread the wonton wrappers, and fill each with a large spoonful of the filling. Wrap the wontons into triangles, so that the wrappers fully cover the filling, and seal with a drop of the water.

4. Coat each filled and wrapped wonton thoroughly with the vegetable oil, to help ensure a nice crispy fry. Place the wontons on the foil-lined air-fryer basket.

5. Set the air fryer oven timer to 25 minutes. Halfway through cooking time, shake the handle of the air fryer basket vigorously to jostle the wontons, and ensure even frying. After 25 minutes, when the air fryer oven shuts off, the wontons will be crispy golden-brown on the outside, juicy, and delicious on the inside. Serve directly from the air fryer basket and enjoy while hot.

Nutrition: Calories 30, Fat 1 g, Carbohydrates 4 g, Protein 0.9 g.

34. CILANTRO-MINT PORK BBQ THAI STYLE

A Perfect Classic Recipe for Pork

 Easy

 15 minutes

 Pork Recipes

 3 Servings

INGREDIENTS

1 minced hot Chile

1 minced shallot

1-pound ground pork

2 tablespoons fish sauce

2 tablespoons lime juice

3 tablespoons basil

tablespoons chopped mint

3 tablespoons cilantro

COOKING STEPS

1. In a shallow dish, mix well all ingredients with hands. Form into 1-inch ovals.

2. Thread ovals in skewers. Place on skewer rack in an air fryer.

3. For 15 minutes, cook at 360°F. Halfway through cooking time, turnover skewers. If needed, cook in batches.

4. Serve and enjoy.

Nutrition: Calories 455, Fat 31 g, Carbohydrates 8 g, Protein 40.9 g.

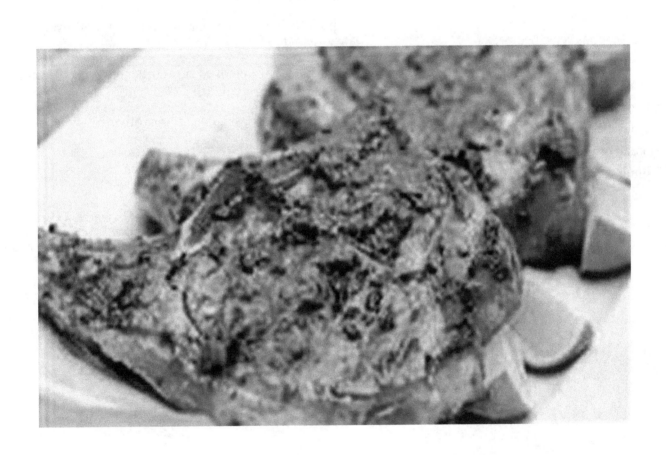

35. TUSCAN PORK CHOPS

A Perfect Classic Recipe for Pork

Easy

10 minutes

Pork Recipes

4 Servings

INGREDIENTS

1/4 cup all-purpose flour

1 teaspoon salt

3/4 teaspoons seasoned pepper

4 (1-inch-thick) boneless pork chops

1 tablespoon olive oil

3 to 4 garlic cloves

1/3 cup balsamic vinegar

1/3 cup chicken broth

3 plum tomatoes, seeded and diced

tablespoons capers

COOKING STEPS

1. Combine flour, salt, and pepper

2. Press pork chops into flour mixture on both sides until evenly covered.

3. Cook in your air fryer oven at 360 degrees for 14 minutes, flipping halfway through.

4. While the pork chops cook, warm olive oil in a medium skillet.

5. Add garlic and sauté for 1 minute; then mix in vinegar and chicken broth.

6. Add capers and tomatoes and turn to high heat.

7. Bring the sauce to a boil, stirring regularly, and then add pork chops, cooking for one minute.

8. Remove from heat and cover for about 5 minutes to allow the pork to absorb some of the sauce; serve hot.

Nutrition: Calories 349, Fat 23 g, Fiber 1.5 g, Protein 20 g.

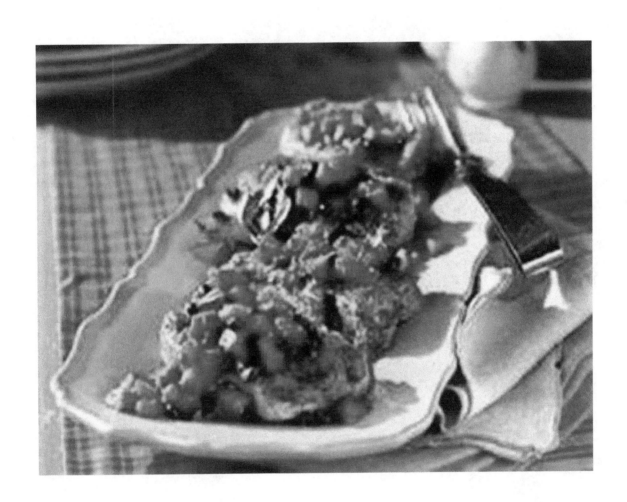

CHAPTER 9: BEEF RECIPES

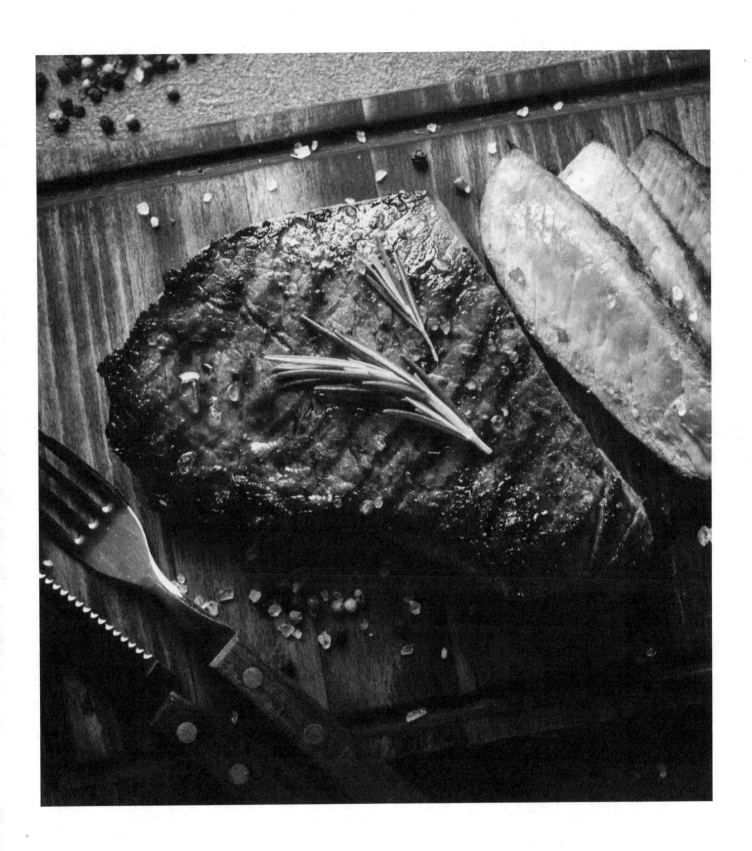

36. SWEDISH MEATBALLS

A Perfect Classic Recipe for Beef

| Easy | 14 minutes | **Beef Recipes** | 4 Servings |

INGREDIENTS

1 pound 93% lean ground beef

1 (1-ounce) packet Lipton Onion Recipe Soup & Dip Mix

⅓ cup bread crumbs

1 egg, beaten

Salt

Pepper

For the gravy

1 cup beef broth

⅓ cup heavy cream

tablespoons all-purpose flour

COOKING STEPS

1. Preparing the Ingredients. In a large bowl, combine the ground beef, onion soup mix, breadcrumbs, egg, and salt and pepper to taste. Mix thoroughly.

2. Using 2 tablespoons of the meat mixture create each meatball by rolling the beef mixture around in your hands. This should yield about 10 meatballs.

3. Air Frying. Place the meatballs in the Air fryer oven. It is okay to stack them. Set temperature to 360°F. Cook for 14 minutes.

4. While the meatballs cook, prepare the gravy. Heat a saucepan over medium-high heat.

5. Add the beef broth and heavy cream. Stir for 1 to 2 minutes.

6. Add the flour and stir. Cover and allow the sauce to simmer for 3 to 4 minutes, or until thick.

7. Drizzle the gravy over the meatballs and serve.

Nutrition: Calories 178, Fat 14 g, Fiber 10 g, Protein 9 g.

37. TENDER BEEF WITH SOUR CREAM SAUCE

A Perfect Classic Recipe for Beef

| Easy | 12 minutes | **Beef Recipes** | 2 Servings |

INGREDIENTS

9 ounces tender beef, chopped

cup scallions, chopped

cloves garlic smashed

3/4 cup sour cream

3/4 teaspoon salt

1/4 teaspoon black pepper, or to taste

1/2 teaspoon dried dill weed

COOKING STEPS

1. Preparing the Ingredients. Add the beef, scallions, and garlic to the baking dish.

2. Air Frying. Cook for about 5 minutes at 390 degrees F.

3. Once the meat is starting to tender, pour in the sour cream. Stir in the salt, black pepper, and dill.

4. Now, cook 7 minutes longer.

Nutrition: Calories 371, Fat 21 g, Carbohydrates 13 g, Protein 30 g.

38. AIR FRYER BURGERS

A Perfect Classic Recipe for Beef

Easy

10 minutes

Beef Recipes

4 Servings

INGREDIENTS

pound lean ground beef

1 tsp. dried parsley

½ tsp. dried oregano

½ tsp. pepper

½ tsp. salt

½ tsp. onion powder

½ tsp. garlic powder

Few drops of liquid smoke

1 tsp. Worcestershire sauce

COOKING STEPS

1. Preparing the Ingredients. Ensure your air fryer is preheated to 350 degrees.

2. Mix all seasonings till combined.

3. Place beef in a bowl and add seasonings. Mix well, but do not overmix.

4. Make four patties from the mixture and using your thumb, making an indent in the center of each patty.

5. Add patties to air fryer rack/basket.

6. Air Frying. Set temperature to 350°F, and set time to 10 minutes, and cook 10 minutes. No need to turn.

Nutrition: Calories 148, Fat 5 g, Sugar 1 g, Protein 24 g.

39. CARROT AND BEEF COCKTAIL BALLS

A Perfect Classic Recipe for Beef

Easy

20 minutes

Beef Recipes

10 Servings

INGREDIENTS

pound ground beef

carrots

red onion, peeled and chopped

cloves garlic

1/2 teaspoon dried rosemary, crushed

1/2 teaspoon dried basil

1 teaspoon dried oregano

1 egg

3/4 cup breadcrumbs

1/2 teaspoon salt

1/2 teaspoon black pepper, or to taste

1 cup plain flour

COOKING STEPS

1. Preparing the Ingredients. Place ground beef in a large bowl. In a food processor, pulse the carrot, onion, and garlic; transfer the vegetable mixture to a large-sized bowl.

2. Then, add the rosemary, basil, oregano, egg, breadcrumbs, salt, and black pepper.

3. Shape the mixture into even balls; refrigerate for about 30 minutes. Roll the balls into the flour.

4. Air Frying. Then, air-fry the balls at 350 degrees F for about 20 minutes, turning occasionally; work with batches. Serve with toothpicks.

Nutrition: Calories 116, Fat 7.8 g, Carbohydrates 0 g, Protein 10 g.

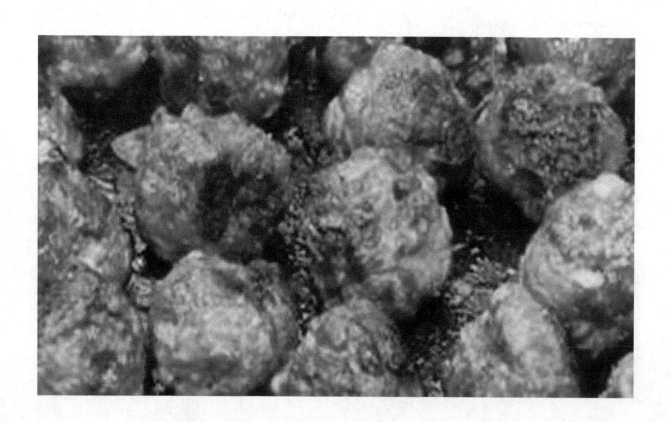

40. BEEF STEAKS WITH BEANS

A Perfect Classic Recipe for Beef

Easy   10 minutes   **Beef Recipes**   4 Servings

INGREDIENTS

4 beef steaks, trim the fat, and cut into strips

cup green onions, chopped

cloves garlic, minced

red bell pepper, seeded and thinly sliced

1 can tomatoes, crushed

1 can cannellini beans

3/4 cup beef broth

1/4 teaspoon dried basil

1/2 teaspoon cayenne pepper

1/2 teaspoon sea salt

1/4 teaspoon ground black pepper, or to taste

COOKING STEPS

1. Preparing the Ingredients. Add the steaks, green onions, and garlic to the Oven rack/basket. Place the Rack on the middle-shelf of the Air fryer oven.

2. Air Frying. Cook at 390 degrees F for 10 minutes, working in batches.

3. Stir in the remaining ingredients and cook for an additional five minutes.

Nutrition: Calories 140, Fat 20 g, Carbohydrates 21 g, Protein 10 g.

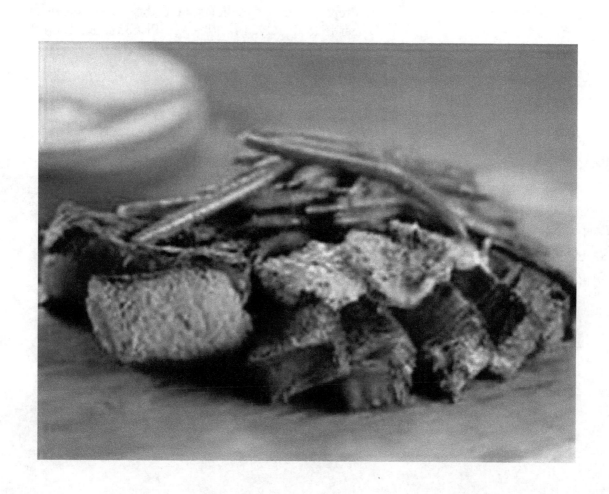

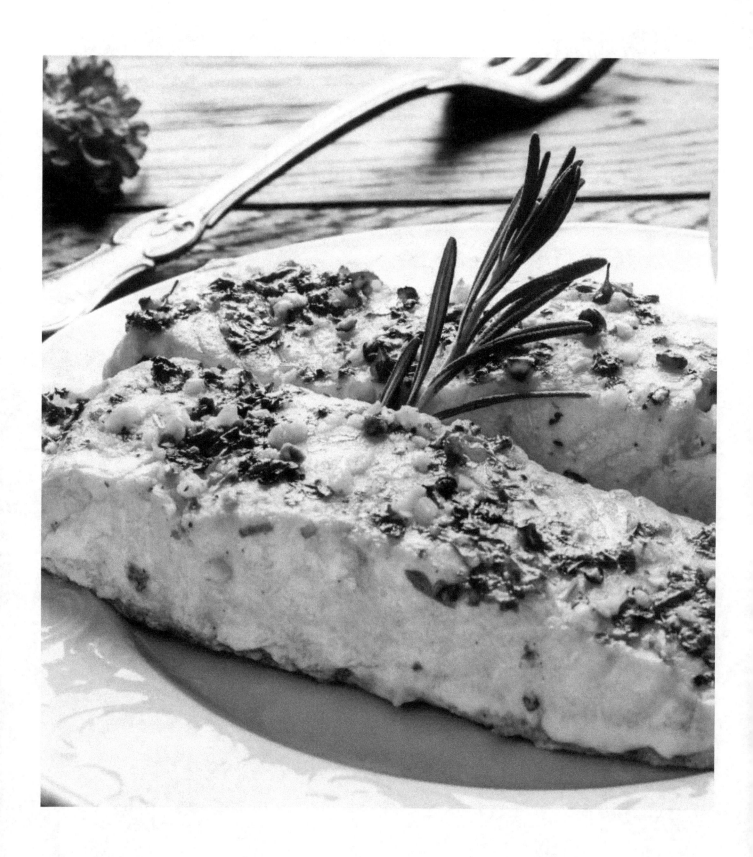

41. FISH AND CAULIFLOWER CAKES

A Perfect Classic Recipe for Fish

Easy

13 minutes

Fish Recipes

4 Servings

INGREDIENTS

1/2 pound cauliflower florets

1/2 teaspoon English mustard

2 tablespoons butter, room temperature

1/2 tablespoon cilantro, minced

2 tablespoons sour cream

2 ½ cups cooked white fish

Salt and freshly cracked black pepper, to savor

COOKING STEPS

1. Boil the cauliflower until tender. Then, purée the cauliflower in your blender. Transfer to a mixing dish.

2. Now, stir in the fish, cilantro, salt, and black pepper.

3. Add the sour cream, English mustard, and butter; mix until everything is well incorporated. Using your hands, shape them into patties.

4. Place in the refrigerator for about 2 hours. Cook for 13 minutes at 395 degrees f. Serve with some extra English mustard.

Nutrition: Calories 285, Fat 15.1 g, Sugar 1.6 g, Carbohydrates 4.3 g, Protein 1.6 g.

42. MARINATED SCALLOPS WITH BUTTER AND BEER

A Perfect Classic Recipe for Fish

| Easy | 1 hour 10 minutes | **Fish Recipes** | 4 Servings |

INGREDIENTS

2 pounds sea scallops

1/2 cup beer

4 tablespoons butter

2 sprigs rosemary, only leaves

Sea salt and freshly cracked black pepper, to taste

COOKING STEPS

1. In a ceramic dish, mix the sea scallops with beer; let it marinate for 1 hour.

2. Meanwhile, preheat your air fryer to 400 degrees f. Melt the butter and add the rosemary leaves. Stir for a few minutes.

3. Discard the marinade and transfer the sea scallops to the air fryer basket. Season with salt and black pepper.

4. Cook the scallops in the preheated air fryer for 7 minutes, shaking the basket halfway through the cooking time. Work in batches.

Nutrition: Calories 471, Fat 27.3 g, Sugar 0.2 g, Carbohydrates 1.9 g, Protein 0.2 g.

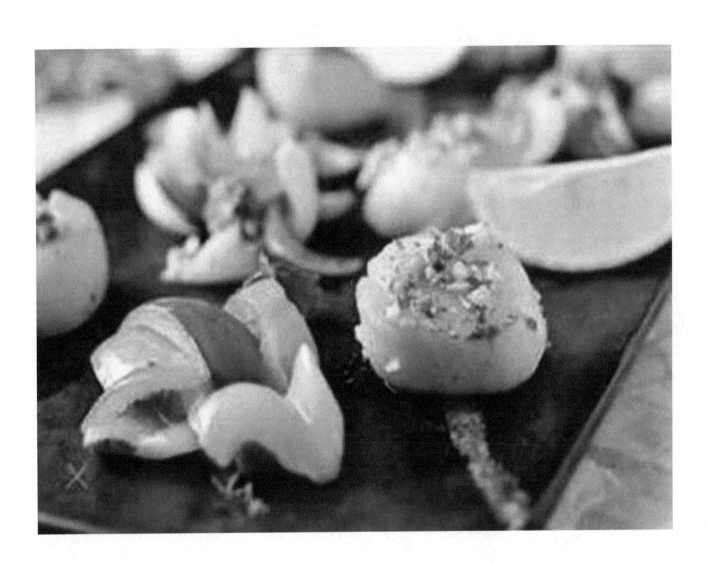

43. CHEESY FISH GRATIN
A Perfect Classic Recipe for Fish

Easy

20 minutes

Fish Recipes

4 Servings

INGREDIENTS

tablespoon avocado oil

1 pound hake fillets

1 teaspoon garlic powder

Sea salt and ground white pepper, to taste

tablespoons shallots, chopped

1 bell pepper, seeded and chopped

1/2 cup cottage cheese

1/2 cup sour cream

1 egg, well whisked

1 teaspoon yellow mustard

1 tablespoon lime juice

1/2 cup Swiss cheese, shredded

COOKING STEPS

1. Brush the bottom and sides of a casserole dish with avocado oil. Add the hake fillets to the casserole dish and sprinkle with garlic powder, salt, and pepper.

2. Add the chopped shallots and bell peppers.

3. In a mixing bowl, thoroughly combine the cottage cheese, sour cream, egg, mustard, and lime juice. Pour the mixture over the fish and spread evenly.

4. Cook in the preheated air fryer at 370 degrees f for 10 minutes.

5. Top with the Swiss cheese and cook an additional 7 minutes. Let it rest for 10 minutes before slicing and serving.

Nutrition: Calories 335, Fat 18.1 g, Sugar 2.6 g, Carbohydrates 7.8 g, Protein 33.7 g.

44. FIJIAN COCONUT FISH

A Perfect Classic Recipe for Fish

Easy

15 minutes

Fish Recipes

2 Servings

INGREDIENTS

cup coconut milk

tablespoons lime juice

tablespoons shoyu sauce

Salt and white pepper, to taste

1 teaspoon turmeric powder

1/2 teaspoon ginger powder

1/2 Thai bird's eye chili, seeded and finely chopped

1 pound tilapia

2 tablespoons olive oil

COOKING STEPS

1. In a mixing bowl, thoroughly combine the coconut milk with the lime juice, shoyu sauce, salt, pepper, turmeric, ginger, and chili pepper. Add tilapia and let it marinate for 1 hour.

2. Brush the air fryer basket with olive oil. Discard the marinade and place the tilapia fillets in the air fryer basket.

3. Cook the tilapia in the preheated air fryer at 400 degrees f for 6 minutes; turn them over and cook for 6 minutes more. Work in batches.

4. Serve with some extra lime wedges if desired.

Nutrition: Calories 426, Fat 21.5 g, Sugar 5 g, Carbohydrates 9.4 g, Protein 50.2 g.

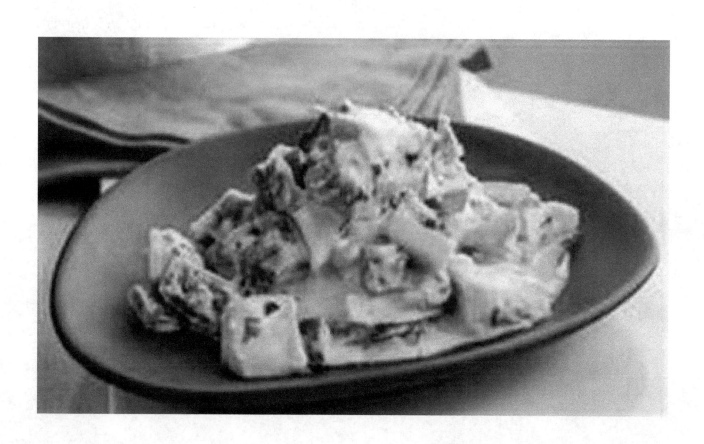

45. SOLE FISH AND CAULIFLOWER FRITTERS

A Perfect Classic Recipe for Fish

Easy · 25 minutes · **Fish Recipes** · 2 Servings

INGREDIENTS

1/2 pound sole fillets

1/2 pound mashed cauliflower

egg, well beaten

1/2 cup red onion, chopped

garlic cloves, minced

tablespoons fresh parsley, chopped

1 bell pepper, finely chopped

1/2 teaspoon scotch bonnet pepper, minced

1 tablespoon olive oil

1 tablespoon coconut aminos

1/2 teaspoon paprika

Salt and white pepper, to taste

COOKING STEPS

1. Start by preheating your air fryer to 395 degrees f. Spritz the sides and bottom of the cooking basket with cooking spray.

2. Cook the sole fillets in the preheated air fryer for 10 minutes, flipping them halfway through the cooking time.

3. In a mixing bowl, mash the sole fillets into flakes. Stir in the remaining ingredients. Shape the fish mixture into patties.

4. Bake in the preheated air fryer at 390 degrees f for 14 minutes, flipping them halfway through the cooking time.

Nutrition: Calories 322, Fat 14 g, Sugar 4.2 g, Carbohydrates 27.4 g, Protein 22.1 g.

CHAPTER 11: DESSERT RECIPES

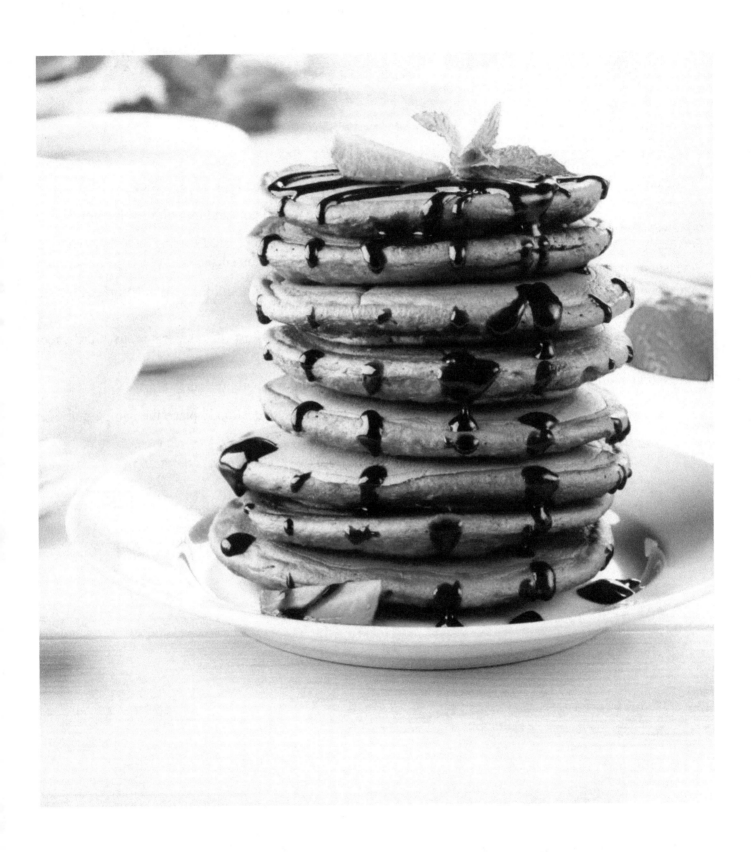

46. CHOCOLATE BROWNIES
A Perfect Classic Recipe for Dessert

Easy

4 minutes

Dessert Recipes

9 Servings

INGREDIENTS

½ cup all-purpose flour

¾ cup sugar

6 tablespoons unsweetened cocoa powder

¼ teaspoon baking powder

¼ teaspoon salt

¼ cup unsalted butter, melted

2 large eggs

tablespoon vegetable oil

½ teaspoon vanilla extract

COOKING STEPS

1. Grease a 7-inch baking pan generously. Set aside.

2. In a bowl, add all the ingredients and mix until well combined.

3. Place the mixture into the prepared baking pan and with the back of a spoon, smooth the top surface.

4. Arrange the drip pan at the bottom of the Instant Vortex Plus Air Fryer Oven cooking chamber.

5. Select "Air Fry" and then adjust the temperature to 330 degrees F.

6. Set the timer for 15 minutes and press the "Start".

7. When the display shows "Add Food" place the baking pan over the drip pan.

8. When the display shows "Turn Food" do nothing.

9. When cooking time is complete, remove the pan from Vortex and place it onto a wire rack to cool completely before cutting.

10. Cut the brownie into desired-sized squares and serve.

Nutrition: Calories 385, Fat 18 g, Fiber 3.1 g, Carbohydrates 54 g, Protein 6.5 g.

47. RUM CAKE
A Perfect Classic Recipe for Dessert

Easy

25 minutes

Dessert Recipes

6 Servings

INGREDIENTS

½ package yellow cake mix
½ (3.4-ounce) package Jell-O instant pudding
2 eggs
¼ cup of vegetable oil
¼ cup of water
¼ cup dark rum

COOKING STEPS

1. In a bowl, add all the ingredients and with an electric mixer, beat until well combined.

2. Arrange a parchment paper in the bottom of a greased 8-inch pan.

3. Now, arrange a foil piece around the cake pan.

4. Place the mixture into the prepared baking pan and with the back of a spoon, smooth the top surface.

5. Arrange the drip pan at the bottom of the Instant Vortex Plus Air Fryer Oven cooking chamber.

6. Select "Air Fry" and then adjust the temperature to 325 degrees F.

7. Set the timer for 25 minutes and press the "Start".

8. When the display shows "Add Food" place the baking pan over the drip pan.

9. When the display shows "Turn Food" do nothing.

10. When cooking time is complete, remove the pan from Vortex and place onto a wire rack to cool for about 10 minutes.

11. Carefully, invert the cake onto a wire rack to cool completely before cutting.

12. Cut into desired-sized slices and serve.

Nutrition: Calories 315, Fat 14.9 g, Fiber 0.4 g, Carbohydrates 36.5 g, Protein 6.5 g.

48. BLUEBERRY COBBLER
A Perfect Classic Recipe for Dessert

Easy	20 minutes	**Dessert Recipes**	6 Servings

INGREDIENTS

2½ cups fresh blueberries

teaspoon vanilla extract

1 teaspoon fresh lemon juice

1 cup of sugar

1 teaspoon flour

1 tablespoon butter, melted

For Topping:

1¾ cups all-purpose flour

6 tablespoons sugar

4 teaspoons baking powder

1 cup milk

5 tablespoons butter

For Sprinkling:

teaspoons sugar

¼ teaspoon ground cinnamon

COOKING STEPS

1. For filling: In a bowl, add all the ingredients and mix until well combined.

2. In another large bowl, mix the flour, baking powder, and sugar.

3. Add the milk and butter and mix until a crumbly mixture forms.

4. For sprinkling: In a small bowl mix the sugar and cinnamon.

5. In the bottom of a greased pan, place the blueberries mixture and top with the flour mixture evenly.

6. Sprinkle the cinnamon sugar on top evenly.

7. Arrange the drip pan at the bottom of the Instant Vortex Plus Air Fryer Oven cooking chamber.

8. Select "Air Fry" and then adjust the temperature to 320 degrees F.

9. Set the timer for 20 minutes and press the "Start".

10. When the display shows "Add Food" place the baking pan over the drip pan.

11. When the display shows "Turn Food" do nothing.

12. When cooking time is complete, remove the pan from Vortex and place onto a wire rack to cool for about 10 minutes before serving.

Nutrition: Calories 459, Fat 12.6 g, Fiber 2.7 g, Carbohydrates 84 g, Protein 5.5 g.

49. SIMPLE & DELICIOUS SPICED APPLES

A Perfect Classic Recipe for Dessert

 Easy

 10 minutes

 Dessert Recipes

 2 Servings

INGREDIENTS

4 apples, sliced

tsp apple pie spice

tbsp. sugar

tbsp. ghee, melted

COOKING STEPS

1. Add apple slices into the mixing bowl. Add remaining ingredients on top of apple slices and toss until well coated.

2. Transfer apple slices on instant vortex air fryer oven pan and air fry at 350 F for 10 minutes.

3. Top with ice cream and serve.

Nutrition: Calories 89, Fat 1.3 g, Fiber 5.3 g, Carbohydrates 21 g, Protein 0.5 g.

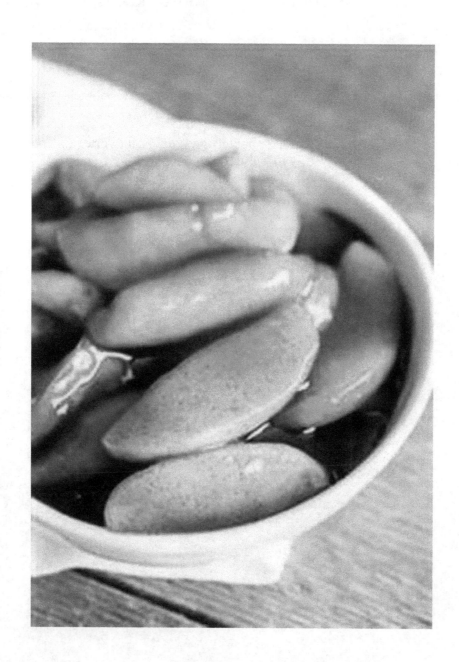

50. DELICIOUS BROWNIES
A Perfect Classic Recipe for Dessert

Easy

33 minutes

Dessert Recipes

2 Servings

INGREDIENTS

2 eggs

½ cup walnuts, chopped

¼ cup all-purpose flour

cup brown sugar

1 ½ tsp vanilla

¼ cup of cocoa powder

½ cup butter

Pinch of salt

COOKING STEPS

1. Spray air fryer shallow baking dish with cooking spray and set aside.

2. In a microwave-safe bowl, combine butter and cocoa powder and microwave until butter is melted. Stir to combine and set aside to cool.

3. Once the butter mixture is cool then whisk in eggs and vanilla.

4. Stir in brown sugar, walnuts, flour, and salt.

5. Pour batter into the prepared baking dish and bake in an instant vortex air fryer oven at 320 F for 33 minutes.

6. Allow to cool completely then slice and serve.

Nutrition: Calories 112, Fat 7 g, Fiber 0 g, Carbohydrates 12 g, Protein 1.5 g.

Conclusion

I hope you enjoyed the recipes you found in this cookbook. I'm sure you've now found that Air Fryer Oven is a useful kitchen appliance that can help you prepare a variety of dishes for your family and friends. Cook delicious breakfasts, juicy meat and poultry dishes, savory seafood, vegetables, and incredible desserts. Thanks to the newest technologies, all your dishes are cooked quickly, they are tasty and useful.

In conclusion, I would like to say Thank You again for buying my cookbook. I am sure that you will return to it again and again in search of tasty and favorite recipes.

CPSIA information can be obtained
at www.ICGtesting.com
Printed in the USA
BVHW011651040521
606415BV00007B/1864